ASK YOUR FAMILY DOCTOR

PRACTICAL GUIDANCE FOR HEALTHY LIVING

David Schechter, M.D.

Ask Your Family Doctor
Practical Guidance for Healthy Living

Includes Bibliographic References
1. General Health 2. Preventive Health 3. Healthcare System
4. Office Visits 5. Nutrition 6. Exercise

Medical Disclaimer
The information presented in this book is intended for educational purposes only. It is not intended to diagnose, treat, cure, or prevent any disease or to provide medical advice for any individual. The author and publisher are not engaged in rendering medical or other professional services to the reader. Reading this book or purchasing it does not establish a physician-patient relationship with the author. Medical decisions should always be made in consultation with your own physician or other qualified healthcare professional, who is familiar with your individual medical history and circumstances. Never disregard professional medical advice or delay seeking it because of information contained in this book.

ISBN: 978-1-929997-04-6 (paperback)
LIbrary of Congress Control Number: 2026918003
First Printing 2026

MindBody Medicine Publications
Contact: publisher@mindbodymedicine.com or 310-836-2225
10780 Santa Monica Blvd., Suite 300, Los Angeles, CA 90025.
www.MindBodyMedicine.com

MINDBODY
MEDICINE
PUBLICATIONS

DEDICATION

I dedicate this book to the tens of thousands of patients who have comprised the 100,000+ patient encounters that I have experienced to date. It has been an honor to be your doctor, whether it was for a half hour or for twenty-five years! Your willingness to share your concerns and your desire to engage with a physician for help has allowed me to serve and to learn…so much. Thank you.

To my family—my wife Lisa, my life partner of over 30 years now. To my sons, Aidan and Noah who have given me a chance to be a father and who do their best to keep me humble. To my friends and colleagues who have supported me and my work.

To my staff who have made it possible for me to be the best physician I can be, with their efforts on behalf of our patients. Healthcare is really a team effort and I've had great members on my team over the years. Especially noted are Cristina and Vanessa.

In memory of my parents, who were surprised when I chose to be a physician, but pleased, as well. Thanks for raising me and giving me the opportunity to pursue my professional interests.

TABLE OF CONTENTS

Introduction: Using the Book vii

Section 1: **Getting Started—the Office Visit** 1
Chapter 1 The Office Visit: Patient History 3
Chapter 2 The Office Visit: Physical Exam 10
Chapter 3 Laboratory Testing and Your Results 17

Section 2: **Lifestyle, Prevention, and Screening** 25
Chapter 4 Nutrition and Diet: Myths and Facts 27
Chapter 5 Exercise and Injury Avoidance 31
Chapter 6 Preventive Care and Cancer Screening 37
Chapter 7 Cardiac Prevention 45
Chapter 8 Genetic Testing: Its Role 49

Section 3: **Optimization and Longevity** 51
Chapter 9 Anti-Aging and Longevity 53
Chapter 10 Sleep Issues: How Sleep Impacts Overall Health ... 57
Chapter 11 Weight Management 61
Chapter 12 Supplements 65

Section 4: **Common Symptoms and Conditions, Part One** 69
Chapter 13 Chronic Pain 71
Chapter 14 Unexplained Symptoms 74
Chapter 15 Headaches 76
Chapter 16 Joint Issues 79
Chapter 17 Digestive Health 87

Chapter 18 The Upper Respiratory Infection: Colds and Flu ... 90

Section 5: Common Symptoms and Conditions, Part Two ... 95
Chapter 19 Urinary Tract Infections ... 97
Chapter 20 Sexually Transmitted Illnesses ... 99
Chapter 21 Erectile Dysfunction ... 102
Chapter 22 Skin Health: Understanding Growths, Moles, and Prevention ... 104
Chapter 23 Mental Health and Stress Management ... 108
Chapter 24 Diabetes Mellitus ... 116
Chapter 25 Thyroid Disease ... 119
Chapter 26 Asthma and COPD ... 121
Chapter 27 Osteoporosis ... 123
Chapter 28 Hormones and Menopause ... 125

Section 6: Medications and Treatments ... 127
Chapter 29 Common Over-the-Counter Medications ... 129
Chapter 30 Common Prescription Medications ... 135
Chapter 31 Alternative Medicine ... 142
Chapter 32 The Preoperative Examination ... 146

Section 7: Navigating Healthcare and Life Stages ... 149
Chapter 33 Navigating the Healthcare System ... 151
Chapter 34 Technology and Health ... 159
Chapter 35 Travel Health ... 162
Chapter 36 Family Planning ... 165
Chapter 37 Workplace Issues ... 168
Chapter 38 Caregiver Support ... 171
Chapter 39 End-of-Life Planning ... 173

Selected Bibliography and Resources ... 177
Topic Finder ... 179

INTRODUCTION

Using the Book

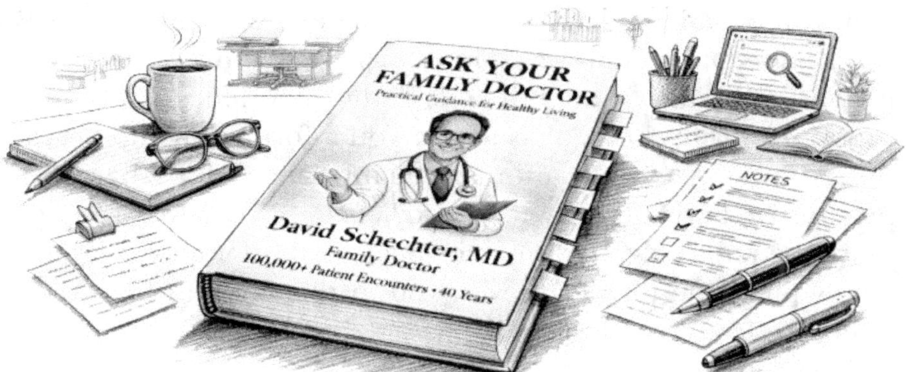

WHY THIS BOOK?

Using this book effectively

This book is for everyone who is sometimes a patient. Being a patient can be challenging, anxiety-provoking, and frustrating. I've been a doctor for many years; forty years or so, but I've also been a patient, so I know from both ends of the experience.

My goal with the book is to give you information and perspective. You can get information on the internet. But it's hard to get perspective and even harder to get wisdom from that source. I share my knowledge and my perspective, that of an experienced family medicine physician, with you in this book to help you be a more effective patient! My style is direct, conversational, and collaborative.

You can read the book straight through, or you can just read chapters that seem relevant and come back to others later. I have divided the book into sections and if you are interested in preparing for an office visit, Section 1 may be most helpful. If you are looking to navigate the healthcare system or end-of-life issues, Section 7 may be a great place to start.

Experience to Share

Since medical school, I have had well over 100,000 patient encounters. That number includes the patients I saw in the hospital and in clinics during residency, as well as years of urgent care and teaching. Most importantly, it includes decades of private practice, seeing new patients, existing patients, old patients, young patients for an incredible variety of concerns and issues.

So I have medical school and residency training and oodles of experience. Some of this learning seems akin to what is now called "machine learning." By this I mean the way computers are trained on huge datasets to answer questions or anticipate problems. I've been trained and developed my skills as a family doctor from this huge data set of patient encounters over decades.

My ongoing learning has been mostly in-office over these years. I learned an enormous amount in my residency program (long hours, long weeks) and an enormous amount more since then. I continue to learn every week. I learn from journals, medical emails, and conferences, but mostly from patient visits—reviewing prior records, specialty notes, and other information patients bring in, and doing brief searches when new problems arise. People continue to fascinate me, and patients have many things in common and many differences as well.

I want to share with you what I regularly discuss with my patients in the office. You don't have to come to the office, meet me, pay a co-pay, or an office-visit fee. You just have to read this book!

Everything I do is customized to the individual patient. But there are many common themes, and that is the essence of what I will share in this book. How does a family doctor with decades of experience answer his patients' questions and direct his patients' care in 2026? I mention the year, because medical knowledge changes and evolves. Some of this information will be different in 2027 and 2028, and a lot will be the same.

More of it will change by 2030 and 2035; that is a certainty. But getting the up-to-date best approaches is going to, by necessity, mean change, and so I hope to update the book in five years or pass this on to another physician-author to do so, at that time. Even as treatments change, the basic principles of medicine and healthcare stay remarkably similar. Lifestyle recommendations don't change as quickly, as well.

I have not written a medical encyclopedia nor a Family Medicine textbook. I do not cover every topic in healthcare; that would be impossible for one author, even a Family Doctor.

Some topics I cover briefly, either because that is all I feel comfortable writing about or because I don't believe you need more information on the subject at this level. This book prepares you to have that conversation with your doctor or doctors that you need to have. Sometimes you find answers to your questions here; other times you discover questions you didn't know you needed to ask of your physician.

For now, it's what I do every day. It's the up-to-date knowledge I have and that I practically apply in my office every week. The book is designed to be conversational in style, evidence-based in fact, and practical for your needs.

Medical students and residents in primary care can benefit from the material and the practical manner in which I present it. There is a lot to learn from these 100,000 visits and decades of reading the medical literature and actually applying it to real-life patients.

Throughout this book, I describe how I think through medical decisions with my patients—but these examples are meant to educate, certainly not replace, the care you receive from your own doctor. Hopefully you'll be better prepared for your doctor visits after reading this book!

Doctor's Note: *Throughout this book, you'll find these "Doctor's Notes" at the end of each chapter. Think of them as the key takeaway I'd give you as you're leaving my office—the essential point distilled into a few sentences. They're meant to reinforce what matters most and give you a clear, actionable perspective on each topic.*

SECTION 1

Getting Started—the Office Visit

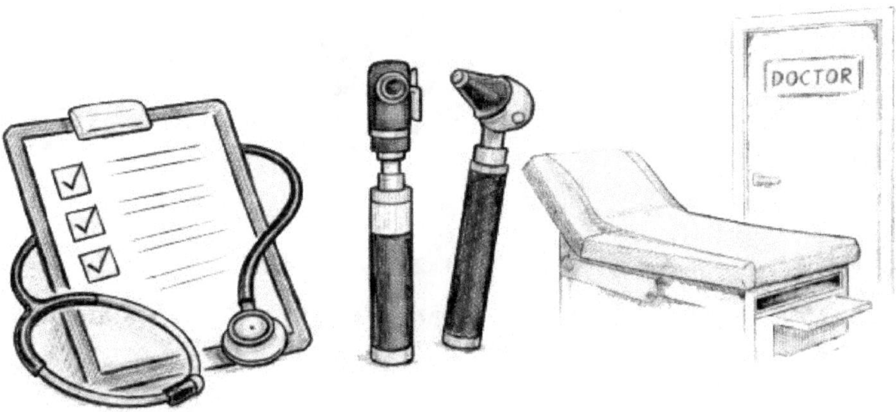

CHAPTER 1

THE OFFICE VISIT: PATIENT HISTORY

We are taught in medical school that the information in the patient history is the key to making the diagnosis. Most of the information we rely upon to make a diagnosis, to direct your care in a personalized way, comes from what you tell the doctor; your "history".

Physicians ask their patients questions about their medical history at the beginning of the visit. Despite this, studies show that doctors interrupt their patients 18 seconds into their initial response. Listening is a key skill for an excellent physician. Make sure you are able to express your concerns early on during the visit to make sure the most important questions are addressed before you leave and there is a plan to address less immediate issues in the future. (see Form at end of this Chapter that helps you to organize your history and thoughts)

One way to make this happen is to prepare some written bullet points for your visit. Whether it is a follow-up visit, where perhaps three issues might be discussed, or an annual comprehensive physical, where the issues might be more preventive or generally focused, including refills, it helps to be prepared. I have, at times, had to negotiate when a patient came in with a list of ten items to discuss. A doctor needs to mentally allocate the time allotted for the visit to the issues that need to be addressed. There are other patients to see that day, after all.

For your first visit with a new physician, or for subsequent visits, be prepared with a family history. That includes a type of genealogy of your parents, siblings, grandparents and specifically their ages and any health conditions they suffer from. Most notably, cancer, heart disease, neurological conditions, dementia, and inherited conditions of all types are relevant.

Be ready with a list of your current medications, ideally typed out or kept in a note on your phone. Either the physician or her assistant will record this medication list in your chart and update it if it is a follow-up visit. If you have had a chance to review the list of medications and allergies in an online medical record summary before the visit, do so. Make a note of any errors or changes you want to make and make sure to inform your physician or the assistant of the needed changes.

Past medical history includes hospitalizations, emergency room visits, any surgeries you have had, and any medical conditions for which you take medications. Again, having that information in a digital format or a neatly written or typed format is very helpful to the doctor and his office staff.

The social history questions include questions about your use of alcohol, cigarettes and other substances. To me, the patient's social history is very important because I work from a biopsychosocial model where the patient's family, home situation, work, and lifestyle is crucial to health and dis-ease. Yes, I want to know, honestly, how much alcohol you drink each week and whether you smoke cigarettes and how much. I do need to document your use of substances including marijuana and cocaine. I also want to know if a patient has used these substances in the past and has stopped. I have had situations where applications for life insurance were denied because the chart record never documented the **discontinuation** of MDMA or cocaine and this created an issue.

Review of systems forms are completed, in my office, prior to the office visit or a physician or assistant may go through a list of symptoms to see if any other relevant issues need to be addressed. Other elements of the history may include a depression screener (see later chapter) or other forms relevant to the chief symptoms.

Lifestyle

Lifestyle is also part of social history. How often do you exercise? What do you do? Do you include resistance training? How often? I am looking to get people started with exercise if they don't currently exercise. If they are active, I encourage them to continue and suggest tweaks where appropriate. People are busy, so advice like making sure you get your exercise before you settle into your home after work may be crucial. Some people go directly from work to a gym or park, others briefly go home to say hello, grab sneakers, and head out the door for a walk or jog. Fine-tuning the right kind of exercise and the right time of day for your lifestyle is crucial.

Exercise or "physical activity" is a really important part of the lifestyle questions I ask. Current recommendations are for 75 minutes or more of moderate to vigorous exercise per week. 150 minutes is even better. That comes out to 30 minutes a day for five days a week. Add in two days of resistance training, body weight exercises, or muscle strengthening workouts and you've reached the recommendations.

But substances are also important. Do you smoke? Do you drink more than a small amount each week? Do you want to cut down? How much? What are the issues for you? Habit? Stress reducer? Socializing? These are common reasons for excessive alcohol or marijuana use.

For men, guidelines advise that 15 or more drinks per week are too much; for women, who tend to be smaller, ten or more. Do you really need that third glass of wine? How about the second? Can you derive pleasure from one glass? These are important matters to discuss as part of a lifestyle assessment and the recommendations that follow. For people with more severe drinking problems, referral to Alcoholics Anonymous or other resources is essential.

I use the social history section to note information about occupation, hobbies, and physical activity/exercise. I also note children's ages and marital status. These are relevant to a patient's health and well-being and represent the environment in which my patient lives and exists outside the office. Also, they allow a minute or two of conversation at the first and subsequent visits that personalize the experience of patient care for my patient, and for me. I learn a little about a lot of occupations in my work and I find people and society fascinating, so that keeps me stimulated and interested.

Patients appreciate that the visit is not just a dry recitation of symptoms and medications. They also understand that some days things are hectic and small talk is more limited.

Doctor's Note: *Your patient history is vital to your physician being able to really understand your health and develop a treatment plan. So be prepared to provide an honest, accurate, and complete history of your health concerns. Show up with any notes the physician may need to review, a list of your medications, your concerns, dates of onset of symptoms and a family history of illness.*

Form to Prepare for Medical Visit

1) Reasons I want to see the doctor: (things bothering me or questions I have)
   a)
   b)
   c)
   d)

____

____

____

2) Medications I take (frequency and dosage)

____

____

____

3) Hospitalizations

____

____

____

4) Surgery I have had

____

____

____

5) Allergies to any medications

____

____

____

6) Age of my parents, if living. Age they died, if deceased. Diseases they had or have or died of (3-4 main ones at most)

____

____

____

7) How often I exercise and what I do. How often I drink alcohol and how much per day or week. If I have ever smoked, how much and for how long. My use of other substances including marijuana, caffeine etc.

____

____

____

8) Dates of preventive tests like mammograms, colonoscopy, pap smear, heart scans, etc. with results (could be simple like normal or polyp, if more complicated, try to bring a report)

____

____

____

CHAPTER 2

THE OFFICE VISIT: PHYSICAL EXAM

I find the most value in a physical examination when there is a specific issue to examine. I have learned from patients that too many doctors skip the physical examination, even in regards to a musculoskeletal complaint. This is concerning. Medical history is important and imaging is valuable, but examination is also very important and may reveal important clues to known and unknown problems. There is also a physician-patient bonding that occurs with being touched as part of an examination that cannot be replaced by staring at an electronic health record, or a virtual visit. Some physicians may skip the examination because of time constraints, a belief it is not important, or they lack skills in examining the part of the body involved (e.g. knee pain).

For the "Annual Physical", the details of what is examined will vary from physician to physician, even among Family Doctors, and depends in part on a patient's age and health status. Physicians always examine the heart and lungs as part of a physical. Lymph nodes should be checked, but how many? Axillary (armpit) and neck are easily done. Inguinal (groin) more often skipped. A breast exam might be appropriate for a female patient, or might be deferred to her gynecologist.

Other important exam areas include: Abdomen, thyroid, and skin. A physical exam of the prostate might be appropriate for a man over forty or with symptoms. But some clinicians use different approaches to evaluating the prostate in an asymptomatic man (for example, the PSA lab test—see later chapter). I usually use both.

When a doctor examines you, he is comparing your neck, axilla, or abdomen to thousands (or tens of thousands) of other patients he has examined since his training began. A doctor looks for something out of the ordinary such as a firm mass, an enlarged liver, unusual lung sounds, etc. Sometimes the doctor can reassure you about something normal. For example, the xiphoid process just under the rib cage in the middle. A couple of times a year a patient comes in asking about noticing a hard structure in that location—and it turns out to be their normal xiphoid process.

Doctors typically examine your facial orifices during a complete exam. The throat may reveal irritation, poor dentition (teeth), or enlarged tonsils. Your neck may reveal a mass or an enlarged thyroid. Usually nothing dangerous or worrisome is found. Comparison by the same doctor from year to year may also detect a change earlier. Some exams lead to a referral to a specialist in that area or to imaging (e.g. CT scan of the abdomen or an ear, nose, and throat doctor (ENT) consultation.

I have been able to find multiple thyroid masses, one thyroid cancer, testicular cancer, and skin cancer on examination, over the years. In some of these cases, the patient had no awareness of an enlargement or change. In other situations, they were curious about something they felt but unsure what it meant.

Whether to do examination of the eye with an ophthalmoscope, whether to do reflex testing of the legs (hitting the front of the knee area with a rubber hammer), whether to check for lesions on the toes, is up to a physician's discretion. Again, this would depend on the patient's health, age, how recently an exam has been done, and many other factors.

But, in general, you should be examined by your doctor!

Vital Signs

Vital Signs are considered part of the physical examination.

The first thing I see in every patient encounter/electronic health record is the patient's name. I have a good memory, so I can usually tell if this is a new patient or an existing patient. My eye is drawn to the chief complaint, the chief reason the patient is coming in that day. My assistant usually gives me a brief synopsis of their preliminary history.

The first thing I notice on the patient's health record after their name and their chief reason for the visit that day are the Vital Signs. These fundamental indicators have been used for some time as a key feature in medical evaluations, both inpatient and in the office. In our electronic health record (EHR), my assistant records height, weight, blood pressure, heart rate, and sometimes temperature. The EHR calculates BMI (body mass index), a shortcut for understanding if the weight fits well with the height.

I learn a lot from the vital signs. Obviously if the blood pressure is high (above 135/85) or even higher (above 145/95), that is important and a focus of the visit. The first blood pressure number listed is the systolic (heart contracts) and the second diastolic (heart relaxes). Both numbers are important. A blood pressure reading is taken by temporarily compressing the artery, usually at the elbow, with a cuff and monitoring the sounds (by ear or now electronically) to determine the pressure at which the blood flow returns to the artery as the cuff releases.

Sometimes the blood pressure is unusually high because the patient rushed through traffic to get to the visit on time. Sometimes it is high because the patient drank coffee too close to the appointment. Sometimes it's a form of an anxious reaction (anticipation rather than reaction) to the doctor's visit called "white coat" hypertension (I haven't worn a white coat in years and neither do my assistants, or most doctors, but the name has stuck). If a blood pressure reading at the beginning of the visit is high, it may be helpful to repeat it again at the end of the visit, after our exam and discussion and when the patient is feeling more settled.

Home Blood Pressure Machines

For a borderline or newly high reading, I may recommend to the patient to purchase a good quality home blood pressure monitor (like ones from Omron, Qardio, iHome, or Hewlett Packard—HP) for $40 to $80 and start measuring blood pressure readings at different times of the day and send me the results. Reports can also occur by bringing in the blood pressure monitor at the next visit (these devices typically store 10–30 readings in memory) or sending me a handmade spreadsheet of readings via the secure online email portal. Some of the more sophisticated machines allow some exporting of data as well.

If blood pressure is high on one occasion and home readings are not great, I have patients come back in for another office measurement. This also includes checking their reading on the machine they purchased against our machine (a $1000+ Welch Allyn monitor). If their machine measures the same as ours, I know to trust the home readings. If not, sometimes it's a technical issue and sometimes they need to replace the machine.

Technique is important: sitting down, placing your arm on a table so that the elbow area (the brachial artery, to be specific) is at the height of one's heart. Too high an arm position, and the reading may be falsely low. Too low an arm position, and a reading may be falsely high. It's best to do a measurement after sitting still for a few minutes. It shouldn't matter which arm, but some people do run higher on one side than the other. Note, that patients have told me that in many offices, the assistants do not have them place their arms on a table and just have them lower their arm. Don't be shy. Ask to place your arm in a fixed place at the level of your heart during a blood pressure reading in the office.

Discussion of the blood pressure may simply consist of obtaining more data and reassessing it. Or it may include recommendations to eat more veggies, follow a Mediterranean diet, consume less salt, and do more cardiovascular (aerobic) exercise. Stress management, meditation, breathing exercises, and sleep may also come up depending on whether this is one aberrant reading or a trend that is calling an alarm.

Weight

Weight is another important vital sign. Is the established patient's weight stable? Have they made progress toward getting to a goal weight? I ask the new patient what they would like to weigh and evaluate that number in relation to height and BMI to see if it's appropriate. Then we discuss getting there. The discussion has typically revolved around the 70/30 rule, a popular simplification that says that "70% of weight loss is dietary and 30% is exercise". The reason for this is that we need a caloric deficit (more calories expended than intake). It is difficult to obtain that with exercise alone unless you are able to exercise at professional athlete levels and durations... which is essentially impossible for nearly all working adults.

So we talk a little about diet and sometimes I have the patient return for additional discussion with an emphasis on lower carb intake. Carbs to avoid include sugar, white rice, white potatoes, white flour, bread. As I discuss later, I also advise limiting carbs for patients with prediabetes. Portion size is another aspect of eating that can require adjustment. For example, a former college athlete, now in a sedentary job, needs to learn to eat much less. A middle-aged individual with a slowing metabolism may need to eat less to maintain weight as he ages.

In this era, for people severely overweight, and especially those with other health issues or who have demonstrated an inability to lose weight, we also discuss the GLP-1 medications. You've heard of Ozempic, Wegovy, Mounjaro, and Zepbound. The former two are semaglutide, the latter two are tirzepatide. They are all brand names, as the category is new and there are no generics available yet. These medications are remarkably effective, typically safe when prescribed and utilized correctly, and pounds come off. But they are expensive, may involve a weekly at-home injection, and titrating results and doses involves follow-up visits, typically monthly, at least at first. (see a later chapter) Also, there are side effects for some people.

Heart Rate

Heart rate is another vital sign. When it's in the usual range, which varies by sex (men tend to be lower) and individually (fitness, size, etc.), I notice the number but it does not lead to conversation. Only when very low (under 50) or quite high (above 90 or 100) does it become a topic. Above 100 can reflect anxiety, but can also be caused by thyroid disease, viral illness, fever, pain, or rarely, a heart issue. Your active heart rate should go above 100; I am referring to resting heart rates while you are seated in the office.

BMI

Body Mass Index (BMI) is a calculated number that is often used to define a normal or healthy range for a person and for society. The number relates to your weight and your height. Here is one of many websites that will calculate it: https://www.calculator.net/bmi-calculator.html

BMI standard measurements are used as markers which determine obesity. Under 25 is considered healthy. 25–27 is borderline or very mildly overweight. 27–30 is overweight. 30–35 is moderately overweight. 35 and above is considered "obese". There are confounding factors. BMI does vary a bit by race. Also, people who are muscular may read falsely high on BMI and be very fit.

The obesity epidemic is defined around BMI values going up in children, adolescents, and adults over the past 50 years. Inactivity, sugar intake, processed foods, video games, and smartphones, all are parceled some blame by many researchers.

Concluding the Office Visit

At the end of the visit, after the history, after the physical examination, perhaps even after your blood is drawn, your doctor should be summarizing, for you and for his notes, the diagnoses and plans.

This is your final chance during the visit to ask for clarification, although notes may be available to you electronically after the visit to review. Also, follow-up visits are a great chance to cover anything that was missed or unclear at this visit. Listen carefully, take notes on paper or your phone, and understand what is planned for you in terms of testing or prescriptions. I encourage patients to take notes in my office because it's hard to otherwise remember all that is discussed in the office visit. I keep on the desk in front of patients a pen and a notepad labelled, "Patient Notepad."

The Annual Physical

Should you even have one? Some healthcare systems discourage them, although most PPO Insurance plans pay annually for a preventive-focused physical, usually without a co-pay. I believe essentially every patient should be seen once a year by a physician. For one thing, if that patient becomes ill, a patient not seen for years by a physician will essentially be unknown to the physician at that time. I do believe in continuity of care and I believe in the relationships that develop with the physician and patient over years of visits. Also, the "Physical" is the best time to delve into preventive care relevant to the individual patient, based upon age, sex, family history, etc. There is never enough time at other visits to go into that depth.

Doctor's Note: *Your doctor should examine the part of your body that hurts or that relates to your presenting symptoms. For a complete physical, more of you should be examined than for a routine visit. Lifestyle should be discussed and the doctor might advise some interventions. You don't need perfection in your lifestyle changes, just steady improvement. Build good habits around sleep, nutrition, movement, and stress management, and you'll be ahead of 90% of people your age.*

CHAPTER 3

Laboratory Testing and Your Results

The first thing to think about regarding lab test results is which lab tests should be ordered for me? This will depend on age, health status, medication usage, and lifestyle. So obviously there are a lot of variations between people.

Common lab tests

The most common lab tests are Complete Blood Count (CBC), Chemistry panel (CMP), Lipid Panel (cholesterol and fats), and Urinalysis.

Let's start with those. On the CBC, I focus upon four numbers. White blood count (leukocytes) is a machine count of how many white blood cells you have per milliliter. Normal range varies per lab, but usually 4–11 or so. It's best to be in the middle or slightly lower. African Americans may be 3–4 and still normal. This points out that lab tests are graded on a curve and the curve depends on which sample of "normals" are used.

Typically, normal is defined as the results that fit under 95% of a bell-shaped curve (reverse U) of all the test results for a particular test in asymptomatic individuals. 2.5% on the low side and 2.5% on the high side are defined as "out of range" and assumed to be abnormal. I say assumed because some of the results at each end are completely normal for that individual. Five percent, or one out of 20 results will, by definition, be considered out of range. So the interpretation is important. That's why I don't like when people order large panels from a lab and await the report results. There is actually quite a bit of knowledge needed to personalize those results for an individual.

CBC

Back to CBC: White blood count is first. Too high—could indicate lab error, an infection, or rarely a blood disease. Too low could indicate lab error, genetic variation, a different type of infection, or a blood condition with reduced immunity. Why lab error? Tests are run semi-automated, and although there is technician supervision, the sample, the machine, the process can fail and result in an error.

The next two numbers I look at are hemoglobin and hematocrit, which together tell us your blood count. Red cells are another aspect of this, but if H and H are fine, usually red blood cell counts are okay as well. Low counts may indicate anemia from blood loss (e.g., gastrointestinal, menstrual, too many donations) and high counts may indicate lab error, a blood condition, or the use of testosterone or other agents that raise red cell counts (such as blood doping—in the Olympics or the Tour de France, the use of Epogen, a medication to raise counts, etc.)

Platelets, Other Values

The fourth is platelet count. Platelets are small cells that help us clot. Normal range is 150 to 450 in many labs. High counts can be lab error or some kind of blood disease. Often slightly high or low counts are monitored for years with nothing alarming showing up. Low counts can be lab error (clumping, for example) or a blood disease where we don't produce enough platelets. Most people are normal in this.

The other values presented in a CBC are sometimes helpful, often not. For example, MCV (mean corpuscular volume) can tell us something about iron deficiency, sickle cell, and other anemias. The differential that includes the type of white cells (eosinophils, lymphocytes, granulocytes, etc.) is helpful in case of infection and rarely otherwise. Small variations in these numbers often alarm patients, and I have answered many questions about "why are my granulocytes two points higher than normal?". One of the keys in lab test evaluations is that very small variations outside of normal range mean far less than larger variations. This goes back to the bell curve and the 2.5% on either side rule that I discussed above. Again, where there are abnormalities, I may retest the patient, perhaps add some additional testing like iron levels or ferritin (iron storage) and see if the abnormalities resolve (e.g. lab error) or if they persist or worsen.

Chemistry Panel

The chemistry panel, or Chem-6, 12, or 24, variations refer to how many tests are included in the automated machine testing of a small sample of your blood. The chemistries look at electrolyte levels (sodium, potassium, chloride, etc.), glucose (sugar), and liver function tests like ALT, AST, bilirubin, etc. Finally, kidney tests as well—blood urea nitrogen (BUN) and creatinine (not creatine). Electrolytes are usually normal or off one from normal, i.e., fine. If there is a substantial variation in a healthy outpatient, I would repeat to rule out lab error. Glucose (sugar) is helpful, but depends upon fasting (normal fasting level under 100, but higher numbers are acceptable after a meal).

Liver tests may show minor or more substantial changes in liver function tests (more accurately, liver cell destruction tests), which can indicate lab error, a viral infection, excessive alcohol use, fatty liver, or something else. I often repeat if abnormal in a few weeks, asking the patient to avoid alcohol for two weeks and skip supplements that may irritate the liver (some are fine like D3 during this process). Interestingly, some of the liver "cleanse" supplements can irritate the liver! I don't advise their use with patients, anyway.

Bilirubin, Kidney tests

Fasting bilirubin is commonly high in a genetic variation called Gilbert's syndrome and is not worrisome. This resolves if you eat before the test! Other liver tests can be ordered as part of this panel or separately (GGTP) if there is more concern. A liver ultrasound may be ordered if liver tests are repeatedly high. If bilirubin is quite high, it could be indicative of liver dysfunction, jaundice, etc. This is rare in healthy outpatients.

Kidney testing is basically the creatinine level, which should be around 1.0. BUN (blood urea nitrogen) (above) can tell me if a patient is on a very high-protein diet (ratio goes up), or dehydrated. Raised creatinine levels can be lab error, related to medications or supplements, or could represent a glitch in kidney function. Further testing might include a 24-hour urine collection for more detailed creatinine analysis, kidney ultrasounds, or a consultation with a specialist in the field. Trends in creatinine can be helpful, as with other lab tests, looking back at a few years' results if available.

Lipid Panel

The lipid panel is something I do focus upon, as well. Total cholesterol is seen first, but is not the most important. Certainly above 200 is a red flag and ideally much lower results are obtained. Next comes HDL, the "good" cholesterol, and generally higher is better here. The ratio of total to HDL is usually given. Four is average and two is superb. Most people are in between. LDL follows, the most important lipid, and "bad" cholesterol number. Guidelines advise patients with repeated LDLs above 160 to be put on medication, regardless of other numbers. But most people are in the 80 to 130 range, where we try to improve this value with exercise, better diet, less red meat and cheese, more fish and vegetables.

Some people do everything right and can't get the LDL down. If there is a family history, this represents a higher risk group that needs prompt attention, with medication and often scanning of the heart to assess risk and disease (see heart screening chapter). Triglycerides are the final lipid value presented in most panels. This one may be more related to simple sugar intake, to carbs in the diet. Fasting levels are typically much lower than those after eating, which is not as true of the other lipids above. Alcohol, a simple sugar, can also raise TGs and high TGs can be a red flag for excessive alcohol use. There can be a genetic element, as well.

Urine Testing

Urinalysis is usually an automated microscopic check combined with a sort of dipstick test. I look for white cells, red cells (erythrocytes), and other elements. The presence of lots of epithelial cells (surface, like skin cells) often indicates the urine catch was not pure enough to evaluate all the cell counts. A culture is ordered if there are symptoms of infection. This takes longer to return, and if bacteria are found, a sensitivity panel may also be provided, guiding antibiotic therapy. UA is the most optional of the above tests in a routine physical, by my assessment. While it may reveal something helpful, it is less likely to, and may have false positive findings, such as red cells after vigorous exercise, or near a woman's menstrual period that can confuse results.

Other Common Lab Tests Ordered

I order a PSA (prostate-specific antigen) for any man over forty years of age. Guidelines have varied, and doing it every other year may be reasonable. However, the opportunity to catch an early-stage prostate cancer, especially in men between 40 and 70, to me, outweighs the cost of the test. Zero to four is usually normal, higher if older, and rapid changes in the values are of great concern. I did find prostate cancer in a man whose PSA was 0.5 every year and jumped to 3.5 (still normal, but quite a leap). I repeated the test to exclude lab error (still just below 4) and sent him to a urologist who diagnosed and treated prostate cancer. Prostate cancer treatment is evolving, and in older men, watchful waiting is often considered. But decisions cannot be made if one doesn't make the initial diagnosis.

HbA1c

Hemoglobin A1c (or HbA1c) is a commonly ordered test to look more precisely than a simple glucose test for diabetes. This test looks at the effects of glucose on red cells over a three-month basis, so one is getting an average value of sugar. Normal is usually 5.6 and below. 5.7–6.4 represents prediabetes, and above 6.5 meets the American Diabetes Association criteria for diabetes. Prediabetes is typically treated, especially initially, with diet and exercise. Diabetes usually needs medication to reduce risks of complications down the line. Overweight people are more prone to prediabetes, although it can occur in anyone. When I see an elevated A1c, it may serve as motivation for my patient to make changes to prevent something more serious in the future.

Hormones

Thyroid function is often tested (see below). Testosterone, estradiol (estrogen), and progesterone can be tested. These are the principal male and female hormones in the body. I will address this more in the hormone section. I focus on testosterone levels in men with symptoms such as reduced energy and vitality, reduced libido, and aging. Three hundred (300) is a cutoff for normal in most guidelines, and the test should be repeated, in the morning, and non-fasting for a second number. Two numbers under 300 meet guidelines to treat; treatment is discussed elsewhere. It's important to point out that men with a testosterone of 320 may feel fantastic with normal or high libido and men with levels of 600 may feel the opposite. Not surprisingly, while our hormones affect us, there is more going on in terms of our energy levels and sexual interest than just these values.

Female hormonal values are even more complicated because they vary with menstrual cycle time of the month. I often rely on a great gynecologist to go over these values in her office.

As noted, some doctors overtest. I don't find value in testing patients for Epstein-Barr virus, other than acute mononucleosis. Lyme disease blood testing is appropriate for someone who had the post-bite rash that is typical of the disease, or rarely for someone with long term concerns about symptoms. Remember that the results are given with many subtypes checked. Typically you need a certain number of positive antibody responses (four in some labs) to be considered a positive (or potentially infected) individual.

STI Testing

STD or STI (sexually transmitted disease or illness) testing is commonly requested and often indicated for individuals who may be approaching or expecting a new sexual relationship or where they are non-monogamous regardless of relationship status. I use a small panel that covers the major areas of concern. An HIV test, testing for HIV 1 and 2, is included. RPR for syphilis is important. Hepatitis C antibody is often ignored, but is another test in this panel. Herpes 1 and 2 are included. Herpes II is typically genital herpes, and one can have antibodies, without obvious prior infection. This brings up a discussion about risks, protection, etc. Herpes I is associated with the cold sore virus.

Herpes 1 is thought to be transmitted from parents to children with kissing and facial contact. While usually non-venereal, oral sex has transmitted the Herpes 1 virus to the genitals of one's partner. Usually this is a one-time event, while genital herpes is more likely to be recurrent. Finally, a urine specimen can be tested for gonorrhea and chlamydia, two common and treatable infections. The lab does an amplified DNA test looking for either of these agents; it is not a culture, and fortunately, a swab of the urethra is no longer necessary (for many years).

Uric Acid

Uric acid is done when there have been high uric acid readings in the past, or for people on a medication to lower uric acid called allopurinol. In addition, while gout cannot be diagnosed by serum uric acid (only by joint aspirated microscopic exam for crystals), an individual with gout whose uric acid is high, can reduce the risk of having more gout attacks by lowering their uric acid.

Thyroid

Thyroid testing is important for weight changes or weight control issues, although in the vast majority of people who are overweight, thyroid function is actually completely normal. This metabolism hormone is not the culprit in most instances. Rapid gain or loss of weight associated with other symptoms may find a thyroid patient (low or high, hypo or hyper). I also check the thyroid function tests of anyone on thyroid medication (levothyroxine or Synthroid, for example). TSH is thyroid-stimulating hormone, a molecule produced in the pituitary gland in response to thyroid levels. T3 is the active form in the body; I usually check free T3. T4 is the precursor, such as the medication's content, that is converted by the body to T3. Free T4 is another option to include.

Doctor's Note: *Lab results are clues, not verdicts. Small variations often mean nothing; trends matter more than single numbers. Understanding your results helps you partner with me in your care—but interpretation requires context and experience.*

SECTION 2

LIFESTYLE, PREVENTION, AND SCREENING

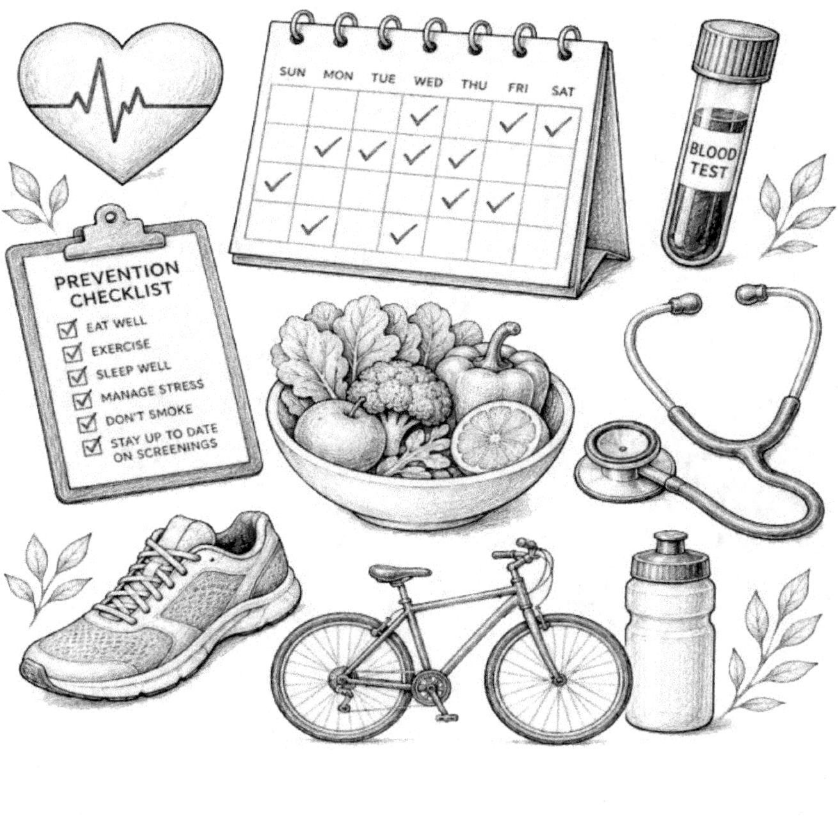

CHAPTER 4

NUTRITION AND DIET: MYTHS AND FACTS

After the preventive visit, the two things I find that I speak about a lot are Nutrition and Diet and Exercise and Activity.

I've learned in my practice and in my life, that different diets work for different people. By this, I am referring to the food people consume, not just a weight loss program. Some people do better with slightly more carbs, others with a more vegetarian approach, and others need more protein. So, again, it's individualized. But there are some common principles and some common misconceptions.

Mediterranean Diet

The diet I advise most commonly is the Mediterranean diet, of which there are various versions and tweaks. This diet is derived from how people eat throughout the Mediterranean region and includes a lot of fresh vegetables and fruits, along with reasonable portions of fish and chicken, some lamb or meat, and herbs, with little added salt. Of the world's diets, this seems to be the most adaptable to most Americans and healthful.

I don't object at all to a healthy version of the South Asian diet. For Americans, this often involves reducing the rice portions and increasing protein a bit. Carbohydrates are an important part of any diet, but for many adults with average metabolisms, too much of the "white foods"—white rice, white potatoes, white bread, etc.—leads to obesity. Why are some people able to eat a very heavily rice-oriented diet and not get overweight in some nations? This may relate to genetic factors, activity level, overall calorie intake, or different food availability. Remember that the diet of the American South was developed in agrarian times. People worked harder and longer than we do at physical labor. Eat this diet and do accounting work, and you will gain weight.

Similarly, most cultures around the world were farming and agriculturally focused and involved a lot more movement and activity than most 21st-century North Americans and Europeans get in their daily routine. So we need to psychologically adjust from what our ancestors and cultures taught us and to what we need to stay fit and at an appropriate weight.

French Paradox

People ask about the "French Paradox" which has been described as the seeming ability of the French to eat more butter, more fatty foods, more red wine, more bread, and not become overweight to the degree that Americans have become. The best explanation I have heard, beyond some genetic differences, is that the French eat fresh ingredients. Bread is baked the same day. Vegetables are sourced more locally. Meat is not fattened up or chemically treated. And meals are relaxed and food is eaten more slowly. Some combination of these factors may explain the French Paradox.

Diet Books

Another phenomenon I have observed over the years has been the publishing of innumerable "diet" books. There was the Beverly Hills Diet, then the Atkins Diet, then the Paleo diet, then the Zone Diet, the South Beach Diet, etc. Why so many diets? For one thing, people want to lose weight, and before the GLP-1 medications (Ozempic, Zepbound, etc.), this was the only real option. Secondly, publishers want to sell books, and apparently diet books sell. Third, different diets work for different people. As noted previously, what works for different people is very different. Someone does well on the Zone Diet, another on Atkins, etc.

Lowering Cholesterol

Many patients need to lower their cholesterol, with the most important value being the LDL (low density lipoprotein). Reducing red meat and cheese is usually helpful. Changing to a more plant-based diet, eating more vegetables, and fish, especially salmon is also beneficial.

Intermittent Fasting

Another approach that is somewhat popular these days is to skip meals, or "fast" for a portion of each day. One common approach is to limit your eating to eight hours a day (10 a.m. to 6 p.m.), for example. Another is to limit further to six hours a day (noon to 6 p.m.). For a subset of the population, this works probably because there are fewer meals and less time to overconsume during these intervals.

Rather than focusing on trendy approaches, I believe in going back to core dietary principles.

First, eat portion sizes appropriate for your body size and activity level—this matters more than any specific food choice.

Second, fill your plate with vegetables and fruit; their health benefits are well-documented.

Third, ensure adequate protein intake, especially as you age—and remember that protein includes beans, nuts, tofu, eggs, and fish, not just meat.

Finally, when in doubt, aim for a colorful plate; our eyes are naturally drawn to variety, and that colorful diversity usually translates to healthy nutrition.

Doctor's Note: *Forget fad diets. Focus on whole foods, vegetables, appropriate portions, and sustainable eating habits you can maintain for life. The Mediterranean diet remains one of the healthiest, most balanced approaches for most people.*

CHAPTER 5

Exercise and Injury Avoidance

As a Family Medicine doctor with additional certification in Sports Medicine, I've seen a lot of injuries and advised on a lot of exercise over the years. In addition, I am an active person myself, quasi-athletic, and have had my share of injuries over the decades.

Finding Time to Exercise

Let's start with exercise. Practicing in Los Angeles, most of my patients drive to work, to groceries, and to entertainment. So focusing on exercise is crucial in this suburban/urban environment that is generally not conducive to walking like parts of New York, Boston, Chicago, or D.C. are. In addition, our mass transit is still developing, and we don't even get the stair climbing or walking to/from buses and trains that people get in some cities. So you must exercise intentionally; it doesn't happen incidentally.

One of the best times of the day to exercise, and this should be individualized, is right after work. For those who go to a gym, directly from work to gym is best, with the gym bag kept in the trunk of one's car. For those who exercise from home, I advise coming home, briefly greeting roommates or spouse or kids, putting exercise shoes on, and getting out. In our mild climate, a brisk walk or run is accessible nearly every day of the year. Once you have sat down and started to engage with others at home or media or mail, it is often much more difficult to shift to exercise mode. This applies to other climates where more exercise needs to be done indoors, depending on the season.

Another time of day that is excellent for some people is early in the morning. This applies to busy executives, working moms, etc. Once the young children are up, it is typically impossible to think about exercise or anything else until they have eaten, been driven to school, and by then you are off to work or other responsibilities. So get up early, and exercise at home or outdoors for at least 30 minutes. Quick shower and you are ready for your day. Some people find it reasonably easy to arise an hour before others and do this. Others do not.

Another possible time to get some activity in—and some is always better than none—is lunch hour. If you have a lunch hour at work, going for a thirty minute walk before eating and then eating is one option. Another option is to at least walk ten minutes to lunch and ten minutes back. We can accumulate exercise and activity minutes all at once or split up. Research shows both to be beneficial. Weekends are another time to get in exercise. It is often easier to get together with a significant other for a walk, run, bike, or hike on the weekends. With young children, the jogging stroller can be pushed while the adults move around flat or up and down hilly areas.

Home exercise equipment can be quite affordable. Start with a basic stationary bicycle if appropriate. Some free weights, even dumbbells, take up very little room.

Building a Positive Exercise Habit

My point in giving these examples is that you need to find the right exercise and the right timing that works for you. Make exercise a positive habit. Become just a bit dependent in that you start feeling better when you do exercise and worse when you miss a couple of days. Different people have different amounts of time and energy to expend and different goals. For some people, two days of brisk walking and two days of tennis are perfect. For others, three days of light jogging and two days of weight or resistance training might be ideal. Some people prefer team activities like volleyball or basketball recreation leagues or pickup games.

The point again, is to find something that you enjoy and works for you. You can listen to podcasts on the treadmill, Peloton, or while walking outdoors if you like. Studies have shown a benefit to walking in nature, even the trees and squirrels in an urban environment. Hearing the breezes or the chirping of birds is probably part of this. Consider one AirPod or equivalent to hear the music or podcast and keep the other ear free for ambient noise. This keeps you more aware of your surroundings, as well.

Exercise improves our mood, fights depression, lowers anxiety and stress. So many benefits in something that is inexpensive or even free.

Include two days of resistance exercise, if possible, good for muscle strength and anti-aging as well. Also, moderate exercise of 150 minutes a week is a reasonable goal based upon the recommendations of national organizations, to stay physically fit.

Injury Avoidance

Along with exercise comes injuries. Hopefully few, far between, and quickly resolved. Certainly injuries take longer to heal with each decade of life. Most ten-year-olds heal really quickly from a bruise, a cut or some roughhousing. Twenty-year-olds heal rapidly. Thirty year olds heal a little slower than at twenty, and so on for each decade. So I emphasize to patients ways to avoid injuries, because the time recovering can set you back and away from your goals for a healthier lifestyle.

One way to accomplish this is with a warm-up. Warm-up is especially important for activities that are competitive or unpredictable. So brisk walking typically requires no formal warm-up. Tennis or pickle ball does, however. Softball does, and table tennis may not. Some of this depends on the intensity at which you play, the competitive nature of the sport (and your competition), and the surface and conditions.

The easiest way to warm-up is to do the planned activity at a slower, more controlled level prior to doing the actual exercise. For example, leaving the house jogging at a 12-minute pace when you run at a 9-minute pace is a good warm-up. Do this for about five minutes, break a light sweat and you are less likely to be injured. For tennis, beginning by running around the court, or to the court, for five minutes can help avoid injury.

Sport-Specific Warm-Up

Sport-specific exercise like shoulder stretching or loosening for tennis may also be of benefit. Serving lightly in practice for ten or twelve serves may get your body ready for full-speed serves during the match. The principle applies to most sports and activities you can think of. Tossing a ball lightly before softball and taking some practice swings with the bat at 50 or 75% effort is a good way to get the muscles, tendons and ligaments ready for the full-speed effort to follow. As a softball player myself, I advise most players over 50 not to sprint full speed to first base after hitting the ball—especially early in the game or in cooler weather; the risk of a hamstring pull exceeds the benefit of possibly beating a close throw to first. I'm competitive, but I also do my best to stay on the field, uninjured. Thankfully I've been fortunate in that regard, in that sport. Some of my teammates are frequently pulling muscles.

General flexibility work like yoga or simple stretching may also make you less likely to pull a muscle or even tear one. But I don't advise vigorous cold stretching. I think the risk of injury from the forceful stretching may exceed the benefit. Get a little warmer first (the five-minute, or break-a-sweat rule) and then stretch more vigorously if you wish. The best time to stretch, from a biomechanical perspective, is after exercise! Your muscles are fully warm, and you can get a nice stretch and I believe allow recovery to be quicker as well. Especially true if you follow the stretch with some good rehydration.

When You Are Hurting

But let's say you hurt the next day, perhaps a calf muscle, lower back, shoulder. What should you do? Some people run to the bottle of NSAIDs (Advil/Aleve), and while this works to reduce the pain and may also reduce inflammation (unlike Tylenol which only works on pain, not inflammation), I'd like to suggest some other options. I do recommend and advise adequate hydration. A dehydrated body seems to recover more slowly from injuries and fatigue. I also advise the use of temperature changes on the area involved. Typically ice is the number one sports medicine injury approach. For back muscle issues, sometimes a hot shower focused on the area, followed by a brief cold pack (contrast therapy) may be ideal.

Healing With Movement

I also suggest very light cardio like a walk to increase blood flow generally. If not tolerated, is there another form of movement you can do? Swimming, stationary bike, or elliptical, and very lightly can be helpful too. Gentle stretching including the affected area can be very helpful in healing. A tennis or lacrosse ball, rubbed against the affected area can help a lot. You can do this on the floor, using body weight to rest on the ball and slowly slide across the area. In some parts of the body, like the upper back, rolling the ball between your body and a door or wall can be easier than it sounds and effective.

Relative Rest

Time and relative rest are the great healers. I say relative rest because for most injuries, total rest is counterproductive and some motion is therapeutic. Movement, in general, is therapeutic. Blood flow increases. Oxygen gets to our tissues better.

There is an arc to healing with minor injuries often hurting more on days 1 and 2 and then receding days 3, 4, and 5. Try to stay positive, even though you are sore and hurt. You can and will heal from most minor mishaps.

When to Seek Help

When the arc of healing is delayed or pauses completely, consider a visit to a physician or physical therapist. Obviously for more severe injuries, with inability to move or an intolerance to touch of the area, urgent care visits can do x-rays if needed and a quicker assessment.

Doctor's Note: *Movement is medicine—whether it's walking quickly around the block, playing a game or training for a 10K. Make activity a daily habit, and listen to your body to stay off the injured list! The benefits—for your body and your mind—are worth it!*

CHAPTER 6

Preventive Care and Cancer Screening

The vital signs are a key element in the office visit, especially one focusing on prevention, like the annual physical. The issue of having a physical each year has become controversial. Some data suggests that patients don't get much yield from a physical and some organizations have stopped doing them. But here's the catch: you only know a patient who comes into the office. Seeing someone every three to five years, who is healthy and relatively young, may be cost-effective, but it is not effective for building a relationship with a doctor, developing trust in the doctor and the office, or having the conversations about prevention and screening that would be missed if visits are only for bronchitis and sprained ankles!

Twenties

Preventive care is very much based upon age and sex. There are specific recommendations from the U.S. Preventive Services Task Force (USPSTF) and various healthcare specialty organizations that mostly agree and overlap. For example, a male in his twenties needs periodic testicular examinations and should consider doing self-exams as well. Both sexes in that decade may need STI screening; women need Pap smears. If you haven't had HPV vaccination in your teens, this is the time to do it. This vaccine helps prevent cervical cancer in women and venereal warts in men and women. Blood pressure checks find the rare individual with a predisposition toward high blood pressure at an early age. Depression screening tests like PHQ-9 (refers to nine questions on this Patient Health Questionnaire) may detect subclinical, borderline, or undiagnosed depression in this age group

Thirties

In one's thirties, preventive guidelines emphasize maintaining a healthy weight, getting immunizations like influenza annually, and checking blood pressure. The latter is called the "silent killer" because without measurement there may be no symptoms until it has progressed to a serious stage. Interestingly, some individuals with high blood pressure, when diagnosed and treated (often with medication, not always) notice fewer headaches and often had not correlated prior headaches with blood pressure (because they were not measuring blood pressure!). Vital signs are helpful regardless of age. STI testing where appropriate is important. Chlamydia can be asymptomatic, especially in women and has fertility risks if untreated. Pap smears may reveal cellular changes that precede cancer that can be treated in the office to prevent a problem down the line. Skin moles may need to be assessed or biopsied (usually removed by shave technique).

Forties

In one's forties, prevention gets more serious. Our risk of disease, especially serious and chronic disease, goes up each decade. Current guidelines are for colonoscopy at age 45 (it was 50 until recently). Data showed that more colon cancers seemed to be happening to younger people so the window was expanded. If a patient has a family history of colon cancer, the age may be five or ten years younger than 45, depending on the age at which the family member had colon cancer and how many relatives have had it. An alternative for individuals who find the colonoscopy process unappealing is Cologuard. This is a lab test which looks for the DNA of colon cancer and advanced polyps in a submitted specimen ("poop in a box") as an alternative. A normal (negative) result means a repeat of this test in three years. A normal colonoscopy usually means 7–10 years before that needs to be repeated. I advise a PSA (prostate specific antigen) test starting at age 40, usually annually. Prostate cancer can occur in one's forties and guidelines are currently ambivalent about early screening. I am not.

More on Colonoscopy

Speaking of colonoscopy: Despite the high anxiety some people have about this procedure, the procedure itself is quite easy because most people are given a simple general anesthetic and sleep through it! Currently propofol is the medication of choice for this and it's often called the best nap you can have. The annoying part of the colonoscopy is therefore not the day of, but the night before, when a prep is done at home. This involves drinking or swallowing a number of substances which lead to an intestinal purge (not painful, but not pleasant) where one repeatedly goes to the toilet, ideally until one's excretions are completely clear. Clear means easy to see through for the doctor doing the test the next morning. These doctors are typically GI doctors (gastroenterologists) although colorectal doctors also do the procedure. A small number of primary care doctors do it as well. I advise colonoscopy strongly, but compromise with ordering the Cologuard test when patients are clearly not going to do the former.

Mammograms

Preventive testing for women revs up with mammograms at around age 40 (sometimes earlier). The mammogram is evolving, with newer technologies to make it more effective and more comfortable. These include 3D mammogram/tomosynthesis and even MRI options. But for many, it still involves the pressing of a hard plate against the breast for images and despite compassionate technicians, it's not a piece of cake. Breast cancer is common and treatment is better, so almost all women choose to do this as advised. Advice varies slightly, but often every two years in the forties and annually thereafter. This should be individualized by your primary care physician or gynecologist. Ultrasound testing can supplement mammography but is not reliable enough to replace it, unfortunately.

Fifties

For men, at around age 50,—sometimes younger,—I advise cardiac preventive screening to begin. There is a whole chapter on this, but I will briefly mention it here. First of all, men are at risk at an earlier age than women for heart disease, for plaque in the coronary arteries. Women get considerable protection from estrogen until that hormone diminishes during menopause and thereafter. Women catch up, but from a lower baseline and therefore heart disease tends to hit a little later in women. For men in their forties going into their fifties, the big three are prostate (PSA testing), colon (colonoscopy) and heart disease (CT scanning). For women, breast (mammography), colon (colonoscopy) and cervical (pap smears). The frequency of PSA testing has been a subject of debate; discuss with your physician.

Optional or Newer Tests

Cancer risk increases with age and the increase is steeper around age 50. Hence some other cancer screening tests may be considered, in this age group, slightly younger, or somewhat older. I am speaking here of blood tests like Galleri (Multi-Cancer Early-Detection or MCED) or body imaging like Prenuvo, Ezra and the like. The Galleri test is a blood test marketed as a multi-cancer early-detection (MCED) test, designed to detect "cancer signals" and provide a prediction about the likely cancer type and where it may be located. Cancers are usually found in earlier, treatable stages. If a signal is detected, additional diagnostic testing is required to confirm whether cancer is present and where it is located. The Galleri test has been studied in large clinical trials showing it can detect cancer signals, though false positives do occur—meaning some people show a cancer signal when no cancer is ultimately found. False negatives also occur, meaning some cancers will not be detected by the test. The evidence base is evolving, and this is a decision best individualized based on risk factors, preferences, and willingness to pursue follow-up testing.

Body Imaging?

Body imaging is even more controversial. Originally done by CT scans, this brought up the issue of radiation exposure and longer-term risks with this modality. Newer body screening imaging is typically MRI which is magnetic; no radiation. The potential benefit is finding a cancer or other problem before symptoms develop, when treatment may be more effective. The major challenge is incidental findings—unexpected abnormalities that are often benign but may trigger follow-up imaging, procedures, cost, and anxiety. The research data on body imaging is still limited, as to its benefit on a population basis. For some patients at higher risk, e.g. a family history of pancreatic cancer, either localized imaging on a regular basis (e.g. MRI/MRCP) or body imaging makes a lot of clinical sense. For others, it may provide peace-of-mind or a baseline scan with which to compare future imaging.

Note that currently, neither of the above testing methods (MCED or body MRI) is covered by most/all health insurance plans. Patients considering these tests should also understand ahead of time that follow-up testing will be recommended if an abnormality or cancer signal is found.

None of these additional tests replace the standard recommendations for cancer screening such as mammogram or colonoscopy.

Vaccinations

- **Influenza shots each fall.** Influenza or flu shots are low risk, effective, and protect you as well as those around you who may be more vulnerable (children, the elderly). Side effects are rare and this is a well-established vaccine, not the mRNA-based technology used for the Covid shots.
- **Tetanus-pertussis boosters every ten years**. The pertussis is whooping cough, which has come back into popularity, so to speak. We get these shots as kids, as teens, but some docs don't check to see if you've had a booster in ten years. I think it's important. It's safe, ultra-low risk, and beneficial. Some people experience a sore arm after the shot for a day or so.
- **Shingles shots** are another consideration for age 50+. Shingles is a skin eruption, a reactivation of the virus that causes chicken pox when you were a child. It hides away for decades and sometimes comes back when we are stressed or older. Vaccinations can reduce the chance of a reactivation and may reduce the severity. For most people, this shot is well tolerated. But, for some people, a fairly significant one to two day flu-like reaction can occur (like Covid shots for some people). Shingles is not a fatal disease, but can be painful, and so I leave this to the patient's discretion after explaining risks and benefits.
- **RSV shots** at age 60 or based upon risk factors (a virus that causes bronchitis and sometimes pneumonia.)
- **Covid shots**—individualized, and will likely change over time.
- **Pneumonia shots**—two types, one-time only. Typically at age 65 or for risk factors sooner. Shots may be given six or more months apart (Prevnar and Pneumovax). Each of these pneumonia vaccines covers different subtypes of this bacterial infection and are well tolerated and significant in preventing serious illness.

Sixties

In one's sixties, the above screening continues—PSA prostate for men, mammograms for women, colonoscopies every 7–10 years for all. Cardiac screening for both sexes. At around 65, recommendations are for a few vaccinations. Two are for pneumonia, which is more common and more serious as we get older. The first vaccine for pneumonia is called Pneumovax and protects a patient against 15 or so strains of bacterial pneumonia. The other is Prevnar, protection against another 9 or so strains. These shots are typically given 6–12 months apart. They are typically one time only so that's good. RSV is a relatively new vaccine that protects against a virus that can cause bronchitis or pneumonia in infants and in older people, more severely. Tdap if more than ten years is also indicated. (tetanus, pertussis)

Flu Facts

Interesting fact: every year, prior to Covid, 40,000 or so Americans died of complications of the flu, often pneumonia. During the Covid pandemic period, fewer people contracted the flu, due to respiratory precautions which worked far better against influenza than they did for Covid. Now that we have relaxed these precautions, the flu has returned. Interestingly, of the four major flu strains, one seems to have completely disappeared during the Covid pandemic!

Flu vaccines are currently including three strains which are predicted to be the active strains for the upcoming winter. Viruses do mutate and may even disappear from the earth. (Smallpox is only found in labs, not in any human or animal population on the earth, as a result of a heavy vaccination campaign and no animal vector in which to hide away)

So to reiterate: flu shots once a year in the fall. Pneumonia vaccines, both six months apart, one time only. RSV shot after 65 or earlier with certain risk factors, one time only. Covid vaccines—people have differences of opinion on this now that Covid appears to be milder than it used to be and most people have a lot of natural immunity from prior infections and booster shots. Higher risk patients should get a booster annually. It may be folded into the flu shot in the future, but not yet.

Aging Out?

Is there an age when preventive screening ends? Some guidelines suggest stopping procedures like Pap smears, mammograms, and colonoscopies at age 75. But I believe this very much depends on patient preference, health status, and life expectancy. If someone is fighting a major illness, a colonoscopy is likely the last thing being considered by the physicians or patient involved.

On the other hand, a physically and mentally healthy 80-year-old may wish to have another colonoscopy (or Cologuard test) or a mammogram after discussion with their physician. PSA testing can be confusing, because low-grade prostate carcinoma seems to be present in men above 85 or 90 on autopsy, even when they die of a completely different cause. The concept of prostate cancer being something you die with, not from, is highly likely if detected at an older age. Prostate evaluations with newer technologies, like MRI scans, can also be used to monitor localized disease to avoid invasive biopsies or other treatments beyond a certain age.

Preventive Care Review

Preventive care isn't just about avoiding illness—it's about optimizing your health, detecting problems early, and keeping your body in good working order for decades to come. Your family doctor is your partner in this process, helping to individualize recommendations based on your age, health, and family and personal risk factors, as well as personal priorities.

> ***Doctor's Note:*** *Prevention is powerful. The right tests at the right times can save your life—so stay informed, and don't skip your screenings.*

CHAPTER 7

CARDIAC PREVENTION

History of EKG testing

This is an important subject and one that evolved over the years. Perhaps 25 years ago, an EKG (electrocardiogram, or ECG) was done on people to evaluate the heart, perhaps starting at age 50. A stress test was performed with higher levels of concern or for executive or pilot physicals. This involves monitored exercise on a treadmill, following a specific protocol, while one's EKG is monitored by a doctor or technician and both symptoms, exercise tolerance, and the tracing are correlated. This approach identified some disease, but it missed a significant amount. It missed disease because it was not directly evaluating the underlying problem—coronary atherosclerosis or plaque—but rather measuring the downstream effects of plaque narrowing arteries and causing ischemia (reduced blood and oxygen flow) of the heart muscle.

The Calcium score

About fifteen or so years ago, calcium score screening was becoming my screening test of choice for heart disease. Calcium scans use CT (computerized tomography) technology, to measure and record the amount of calcium in the coronary arteries. Calcium is seen in plaque, and this gave us a more precise count on the amount of calcified, or "hard" plaque in the arteries. Studies began to show a relationship between calcium score and heart attack risk, and this was more precise than stress testing or the EKG test.

Coronary CT Angiogram

In the last five to eight years, cardiac CT angiogram has become my test of choice for heart disease screening and evaluation. The reason is that this test, done with a small dye injection and a gated scan of the coronary arteries as the dye passes through these vital vessels that supply blood to the heart, measures hard and soft plaque. I individualize my decision based upon patient preference, cost, cholesterol levels and family history. Some choose a calcium scan instead, which is less expensive and involves no dye injection, which is important if there is a dye allergy.

Research has shown that it's better not to have any plaque, but soft plaque is riskier, because it appears to have a higher chance of rupture than hard plaque. So calcified plaque is typically stable plaque. Converting soft plaque, where present, to hard plaque actually benefits the patient. Stopping plaque progression, and where possible, reducing plaque is of course, the ultimate path to reducing heart attacks and cardiac-related deaths.

But before you can intervene, you must detect and define heart disease. These scans, using CT technology, have become less expensive and use less radiation than they did eight or so years ago and can be repeated, where appropriate, in one to five years to monitor progress.

Who Should be Screened?

Back to screening—First of all, who should be screened?

I start with the higher-risk individuals. In this category, I include all men aged 50 or older who haven't had it done. Women at age 60 fall into a similar risk category. Women develop coronary disease later than men due to the preventive benefit of estrogen on vascular disease. Of course, during menopause, estrogen diminishes dramatically and women begin to increase their risk. The role of hormone replacement is not totally understood here, but may delay heart disease further. These age decisions are modified based upon family history and other risk factors, or early menopause, for example, without hormone replacement.

Another higher-risk group is those with a family history of heart disease. I ask men (the higher risk to begin with) in their thirties and forties if there is a family history of heart disease, especially at a younger age, in their fathers, uncles, and the like. A first-degree relative (like parents and siblings) who had a bypass operation before age 60 will prompt me to suggest a CT angiogram at age 40, rather than 50. This should be individualized. High cholesterol or specifically high LDL cholesterol levels may also necessitate more aggressive imaging in terms of age of first test and sometimes frequency of testing.

Earlier screening may be appropriate if you:

- Have a first-degree relative with early heart disease (e.g., bypass surgery before age 60)
- Have high LDL cholesterol—especially above 140
- Have multiple risk factors (e.g., hypertension, smoking, diabetes)

Evaluating Results

In case you are curious, and I am sure you are, the results of the CT angiogram, along with family history, along with LDL cholesterol numbers, leads to an individualized decision to begin medication. Usually a statin (atorvastatin/Lipitor or rosuvastatin/Crestor, my favorites) is the first choice. Sometimes this is combined with ezetimibe/Zetia for further lowering, Often low-dose aspirin at 81 mg is advised along with the statin. I don't ignore lifestyle and diet here, but once plaque has developed, I believe it is appropriate to go to medication in addition to lifestyle. Lifestyle and diet alone seem very appropriate for people in their forties with high cholesterol readings and other risk factors.

Calcium Score

Usually a calcium score comes with the CT angiogram, so I get two sets of data to work with. A relatively low calcium score with mixed or soft plaque is of concern, because the soft plaque is higher risk for rupture and heart attack than is more stable, hard plaque. Treatment goals include low LDL levels (30–45 range) and converting soft to hard plaque over a period of years. These LDL goals may seem aggressive to you if you were taught that 70 is a great number and 90 is okay. Current cardiology approaches support very low LDL goals (30–45 range) for patients with known arterial plaque, as research shows that "lower is better" when it comes to preventing heart attacks in these higher-risk patients.

The best heart disease screening doesn't just look for blockages—it helps us get ahead of them. With today's technology, we can spot plaque earlier, target high-risk individuals, and take action to prevent heart attacks before they happen. That's the real power of cardiac screening in modern medicine.

> **Doctor's Note:** *Know your numbers—blood pressure, cholesterol, glucose—and act early. Heart disease prevention starts decades before the first symptom.*

CHAPTER 8
GENETIC TESTING: ITS ROLE

Genetic or genomic medicine is rapidly advancing. Eventually, it would be ideal to organize our preventive care for patients based upon their biological risks, rather than just family history or age and sex. We are not there yet, but genetic testing is progressing.

Do I recommend my patients get genetic testing routinely? Until the recent bankruptcy of 23andMe, I found that company to be a reasonable option for patients who wanted to know their risk factors for various diseases. Many had no risks or minor increases in the risk for diabetes, heart disease, etc. Some had genetic cancer risks like BRCA (BRCA1, BRCA2) picked up on this testing. This leads to more actionable testing or other procedures, depending on age and sex.

There are other companies doing this type of testing, and I want to clearly differentiate this from "ancestry" testing, which is more for curiosity about the past than it is about understanding health risks for the future. I would say the results have not typically been "actionable" so I don't do this routinely on my patients.

In more complicated cases, with extensive or unusual family histories of illness, I will refer a patient to a local hospital that has great genetic counselors in their genetics department. These individuals can advise my patients on the most appropriate testing and the latest risk factor analyses for cancer and other disorders. This field is growing rapidly.

Genetic testing can be done to help determine the best choice for an antidepressant in an individual, or to look for medications that may not work as well in that patient. The results of this testing, to date, have been disappointing to me. They have not proven to be more effective than clinical choice of medication, or "trial and error" changes in medications. Again, this may change in the near or distant future.

Doctor's Note: *Genetic testing can reveal important health risks—like BRCA genes for cancer—that change how we screen and prevent disease. But it's different from ancestry testing. If you have a significant family history of disease, genetic counseling may be worth exploring. Clinical genetic testing is often clearer and more detailed than consumer genomic testing.*

SECTION 3

Optimization and Longevity

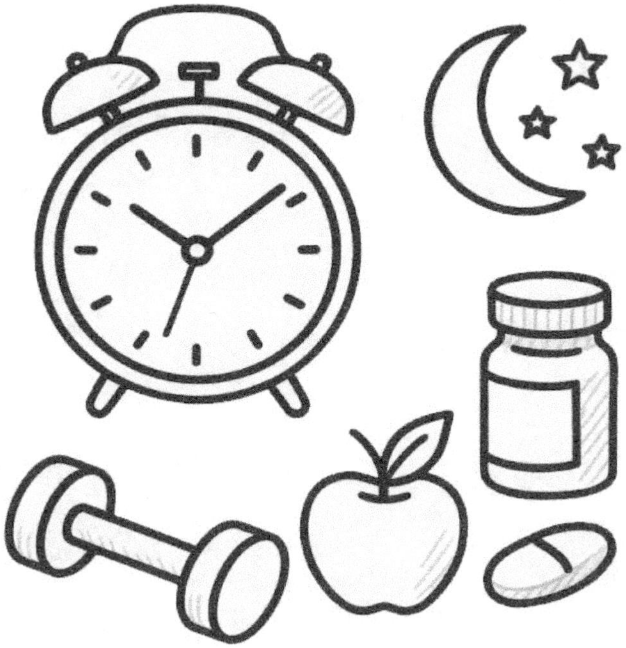

CHAPTER 9

ANTI-AGING AND LONGEVITY

People ask me about supplements and treatments to slow down the aging process. There is plenty of information online and quite a few books on this subject appear every year. Sometimes the supplements my patient is taking prompt me to ask how the information was obtained. As you can imagine, some of the articles online are accurate and scientific, and many are hyped up or inaccurate. So this discussion may involve a longer conversation about expectations, evidence, and priorities

The Basics

My first advice to people on the subject of anti-aging is that, before you delve into the newer, additional approaches, start with the basics. We know a lot about the basics of anti-aging. One key is exercise. Are you getting enough exercise in frequency and intensity? While all exercise and movement is beneficial, some anti-aging research suggests that intense exercise is of more benefit. So start with exercise, if you want to grow old more gracefully and have a longer lifespan and healthspan. It is good for your body, your brain, and your longevity.

Healthspan

Healthspan is the concept of how long you are healthy, rather than focusing exclusively on the length of one's life. Most people would choose an 84-year healthspan with an 86-year lifespan, rather than an 80-year healthspan with a 90-year lifespan. We want to be able to move, to think, to interact with others as we age. We don't want to survive; we want to be as healthy as possible for as long as possible. We want to stay engaged as long as we can.

Nutrition

After exercise, nutrition. Are you eating a healthy diet? Are you getting those crucial servings of vegetables and fruits that have the antioxidants and anti-inflammatory nutrients we need to age slowly? The well-known Mediterranean diet is an example of an overall eating approach that fosters health and healthspan. Many elements of the Asian diet are also conducive to healthy aging as well. Avoid processed foods as much as possible. Things that are boxed on the shelf with a long expiration date may not be healthy for you.

Blue Zones

Are you familiar with the Blue Zones? Researchers have identified certain areas of the planet where people seem to live longer than other communities. They have also analyzed why this may be the case and in some instances noticed changes as lifestyle gradually has become more modernized or Westernized. One of the Blue Zones is in the US—Loma Linda, California. This community has many Seventh-Day Adventists who focus on a vegetarian diet, exercise, and social support in their lifestyles. Sardinia is a Mediterranean island with longer healthspans. People walk a lot, eat fresh food, and often are friends with their elementary school classmates their entire lives. The Japanese island of Okinawa is another. Many similarities are seen in activity level, types of food (beans, vegetables, limited meat, more fish) in several of these

Blue Zone communities. Commonalities include plant-focused diets, strong social ties, stress reduction practices, and a sense of purpose, even in later life.

Sleep

After nutrition, I would emphasize sleep. Make sure you get enough sleep to be well rested. Research supports going to sleep at the same time and getting up at about the same time as often as possible. Sleeping in a cooler, dark room, or using eye shades may lead to more deep sleep. Sleep is when we recover from the day's activities physically and psychologically. Our body and our brain recover. The brain needs good sleep to flush out its own waste products and refresh for the upcoming day. Try to get quality sleep as often as you can. In some ways this is easier as we begin to age, because childcare responsibilities and work responsibilities may be absent or more flexible as we get older.

Core Principles

Exercise. Nutrition. Sleep. Social Engagement. These core principles of a healthy lifestyle are also core factors in anti-aging. Do these things and then worry about the newest research in supplements or other co-factors that may help your aging process. This I believe, and this I share with my patients. Go to the basics first.

Supplements

What is currently interesting in the supplement area for anti-aging? Resveratrol is a compound found in red wine and some berries, and NAD precursors like NMN and NR are commonly discussed. These have shown some promise in lab research, but the clinical evidence in humans is still developing. I'm intrigued but cautious. Explore supplements and other therapies once you've built that solid foundation—but remember that science still favors the basics. This will lead to maximizing your healthspan!

Supplement Quality

One factor for people to always consider is that the quality of supplements varies a lot. Studies have shown that from one manufacturer to another, the actual quantity of the desired supplement can vary from the amount stated on the bottle (100%) to none! Even within a manufacturer, there is variation. The supplement industry is not closely monitored by the FDA, which inspects pharmaceutical manufacturing plants every year or two worldwide. There is no relevant supervision in the supplement field. Buying a well-known brand may help. Paying more for your product may help, but who knows?

Doctor's Note: *Anti-aging isn't about the magic pill—it's about mastering the fundamentals. Start with what we know works: regular exercise, a whole-foods diet, and restorative sleep. These three pillars will support not just a longer life, but a richer, more vibrant one. Research from the Blue Zones can teach us quite a bit about lifestyle in the broader sense, and our health and longevity.*

CHAPTER 10

SLEEP ISSUES: HOW SLEEP IMPACTS OVERALL HEALTH

Lots of people have trouble sleeping. First I start by trying to understand what is the problem—falling asleep, staying asleep, early morning awakening? Is it every night, twice a week, or situational (like travel). A recent problem or lifelong?

Basic Interventions

The ideal treatment is a behavioral intervention. This might include one or more of the following. No caffeine after noon (or 4 p.m. or 10 a.m.), depending on the person. No bright screens after 10 pm (Kindle is an exception; it doesn't produce the same backlighting as phone or TV). Earlier evening meals and avoiding alcohol help some people. Warm milk helps some.

The bedtime ritual is important—the activities that precede going to bed. Some people do very light yoga or tai chi. Others prefer a warm shower. Reading can be a great transition to going to sleep. Going into bed only when tired is another. Unwinding in the late evening is an important part of this. Don't focus on work tasks and worry about what you didn't accomplish that day. These eat up quality sleep.

There is a lot online, books, and now even an online company that helps with cognitive-behavioral approaches to sleep. (The company is Moona.health; there may be more by the time this is published.)

Melatonin is the safest and best over-the-counter option for sleep. A hormone produced in the body, it has been synthesized and can be taken in low dosages and does not require a prescription. Dosages are typically one to three milligrams. Some people who fall asleep but can't stay asleep benefit from a compounded or regular version of melatonin that has extended release (or sustained release) properties or formulation. This means the active ingredient doesn't get absorbed all at once; part of it takes hours to get into your system.

Medication Options

I may discuss medication as one option or one aspect of sleep management. Beyond melatonin, my current go-to would be a prescription for trazodone in 25 or 50 mg. This is an older antidepressant that raises serotonin in the nervous system. In much higher doses it was used for depression, although more recent medications are better and safer for this purpose. But at low dosages, it is a non-addictive, non-benzodiazepine, non-Z drug alternative to fall asleep.

Benzodiazepines are a category of sedative-hypnotic medications used for anxiety, mild anesthesia, and sometimes for sleep. They include diazepam (Valium), lorazepam (Ativan) and clonazepam (Klonopin). They are effective but quite habit forming; easier to get on than to get off. So we try to avoid getting patients started on them. I will prescribe these medications for occasional use such as airplane travel, where a combination of anti-anxiety and sleep properties can be very effective and the usage is so intermittent that no habit is developed.

Z-drugs are zolpidem (Ambien) and zopiclone (Lunesta), zaleplon (Sonata), and related medications. These are also effective;

with Ambien being the most effective, but very habit forming (addictive). For a single night at a hotel, or adjusting time zones, zolpidem is the best. Melatonin is good, too, and many people do fine without anything. Jet lag is handled by the Aussies, who travel around the world more than any other national group I know of, by staying awake in their destination until at least 9 p.m. the first night, regardless of how long they have been up. By the next day, the reset is happening, especially with early morning sun exposure.

Other Medications

Another medication option that is non-addictive and reasonably effective is gabapentin. This medication was developed as an anti-seizure medication but has been found to have many other therapeutic properties. These range from mood stabilizing, nerve pain controlling, and others. A side effect is sleepiness. So we take advantage of that and its mildly anti-anxiety effects by using it before bedtime A dose of 100 mg in older folks, to start, and 300 mg in younger or larger people The dosage can be pushed higher if the individual fails to sleep well and has no morning sedation or other side effects from the medication.

Another older standby is amitriptyline. It is an older tricyclic antidepressant, no longer used for that purpose. At low doses of 10 mg or sometimes 20 mg, it can be sleep inducing, is safe to take daily, and usually wears off before the morning. If a.m. sleepiness is an issue with any of the above medications, taking them an hour earlier in the evening may solve the issue. Used with caution in people above 70 years of age.

Sleep Apnea

Sleep apnea is not snoring although they can go together. It is a medical condition, most commonly obstructive, and most commonly in men with thicker necks. Associated with the relaxation of throat structures with sleep, a mild obstruction of the airway occurs which can be associated with gasping and choking. Sometimes the main symptom is daytime drowsiness. If a patient, usually male, often a little overweight, has these symptoms, they can be tested for this condition. The test used to involve a sleep lab and now can be done in your own home, in your own bed. Results are read by a sleep specialist and sent to your family doctor.

One key treatment for sleep apnea is CPAP (continuous positive airway pressure) although the newer technology is called AUTO-PAP (automatic pressure adjustment) which allows for a simpler process of adjustment. The technology has also gotten smaller, less noisy, more portable, and less obtrusive than it used to be. Patients who get CPAP for a diagnosis of obstructive sleep apnea report sleep better and awakening more rested. The extra oxygen in one's system is likely the reason. Some people even lose weight on this technology. Losing weight may help eliminate sleep apnea, however it is accomplished.

Doctor's Note: *Good sleep isn't a luxury—it's essential medicine. Start with habits: routine, darkness, no screens. If you need medication, use it wisely and temporarily. The goal is always to sleep naturally.*

CHAPTER 11

Weight Management

This is one of the major concerns that patients have and that I have as their family doctor. We spoke about vital signs earlier. Blood pressure, heart rate, sometimes temperature, height, and weight. We can tell a lot about a patient's health status, risk for illness, and even emotional state from the above.

Weight is a big one, so to speak. Most patients with weight issues have tried numerous approaches over the years. Diets, sometimes Weight Watchers, sometimes online apps (Noom is one I like). Some are curious about the GLP-1 medications like Ozempic and Mounjaro.

Let's start with the natural approach. Losing weight should involve more expenditure of calories than input. Output is our metabolism, based upon resting use of calories and active use of calories. Activity is important and it's more than just exercise in the traditional sense. One study described people who are slimmer as more fidgety on video observation. Even these small movements burn calories, and over the course of the day, can burn quite a few.

70/30 Rule

Some experts have suggested that 70% of weight loss is dietary, 30% is exercise. The reason for this, I believe, is that we can't train like Olympic athletes, four to six hours a day, and we are not hunter-gatherers, walking ten to twelve hours a day to collect food. So we are left with revving our metabolism with activity, but focusing on our intake. Many of my patients do well, at least for a while, with caloric restriction.

More often than not, patients do well by restricting the excessive carbohydrates in their diet. This means cutting down, or out, bread, white rice, pasta, and white potatoes. Moderate amounts of complex carbs like oatmeal, brown rice, and sweet potatoes, are usually tolerated—in moderation. This reduces calories and I encourage patients to include healthy fats like avocados, olive oil, and the like. Lots of lean protein, especially fish, as well.

I have had patients lose 70–100 pounds with this formula, but many lose none, some gain it all back. A sustainable change in diet is what I advise, not a short-term "diet". Sustainable in this case means that you must learn to eat in a way that you can eat for the rest of your life. That is the only way to stay leaner once you've lost a considerable amount of weight.

GLP-1 Medications (e.g., Ozempic)

On to GLP-1 medications. I discuss GLP-1 medications with patients who have struggled despite lifestyle efforts. While initially skeptical, I have found the majority of patients who take these medications lose substantial amounts of weight, usually with minimal or no side effects. Cravings are dramatically reduced for sweets, for larger portions, and even for alcohol! Again, the principle of starting at a low dose is important. I start almost all of my patients on this medication at the lowest dose for the particular medication (Ozempic, Wegovy, Mounjaro, Zepbound). All are currently injections, administered by the patient once a week. People find it easy to do with the prefilled pen.

People eat less, crave less, and lose weight. I adjust the medication dosage upwards when weight loss seems to plateau or slow down. GLP-1 medications are very effective for weight loss and reduce cravings. Recent large studies have shown cardiovascular benefits beyond weight loss, and ongoing research is exploring other potential benefits including effects on inflammation and kidney health.

The biggest issue with these medications is cost. Some insurance companies cover it for obesity. Most cover these medications for diabetes. Some insurance companies cover it for being overweight if you've had a six-month supervised medical program of weight loss (dietician, apps, etc.). Others won't cover it at all. Retail costs were initially very high, above $1000 per month. Recently, costs have dropped, especially when ordered by the physician from the manufacturer's pharmacy to the patient (e.g. Lilly Direct Self Pay Pharmacy). This is still a lot of money for most patients, even with the amazing effects. Even more discounts have come along, including ordering directly from the manufacturer.

Forever Meds?

Do you have to take these meds forever? This is a fascinating question as we are still in the early stages of using these medications. I have had patients successfully space out the use of these meds from weekly to ten days, to two weeks, and eventually stop completely. I emphasize to them that they must use the knowledge gained of how a 200-pound person eats to keep eating that amount. If you eat like a 280-lb person, you will return to 280 pounds.

Development of a less expensive oral version of the medication that has been tested and can be used for longer periods, or indefinitely is another pathway forward. Experts point out that people with hypertension (high blood pressure) take their meds for life in most cases. Why not apply the same approach to those with substantial, often lifelong obesity issues? For those with diabetes, there is a double benefit of great sugar control AND weight loss, and insurance is more forgiving in these cases.

These medications seem to act on willpower, metabolism, and cravings. If a patient can develop these abilities on their own, and use exercise to rev metabolism, they may be successful at getting off the medications and not needing them again. Each individual has different needs, and time will tell on these relatively new medications.

Do Diets Work?

Fad diets don't work or are temporary, and people may yo-yo with weight loss, which is not healthy. Truly changing one's approach to eating, one's portion sizes, and food choices can create a sustainable, lifelong weight reduction toward the normal range. GLP-1 medications are very effective for weight loss, reduce cravings, may have other benefits, but are expensive and may be needed indefinitely in some people.

Doctor's Note: *Sustainable weight loss is about changing how you eat for life, not following a temporary diet. GLP-1 medications are powerful tools, but they work best combined with lasting lifestyle changes. Focus on the 70/30 rule: dietary intake matters most.*

CHAPTER 12
SUPPLEMENTS

Most recent scientific research has emphasized that the best way to get nutrients is through food, not supplements. This goes along with the saying that Americans have the most expensive urine in the world because we are excreting so many vitamins and minerals that we take in addition to our abundant food supply. I concur that the best way to get nutrition and nutrients is from food.

Ideal Supplement

So what would be the ideal supplement? I believe it is a substance we can measure in the blood and determine specifically if a patient is low, advise a particular dosage to take, and re-measure the blood level at a logical interval. And the supplement would have known benefits when corrected from deficient to normal levels.

Does this exist? Yes. Also, there are many supplements that do not meet this ideal criterion.

First of all, the ideal category. One that comes to mind easily is Vitamin B12 also known as cyanocobalamin. Easily measurable, supplemented by oral, sublingual (under the tongue) or injectable methods. It is easy to determine if it is back to normal range. Also, it has some clear correlation—if too low—with cognitive and neurological symptoms and risks in certain people. People at risk include vegans and the elderly.

Vitamin D3

Another that is close to ideal is Vitamin D3. Easy to measure, easy to supplement. Most people can correct to the normal range, and there is a wide range of blood levels believed to be safe. Studies have varied a bit, with some suggesting major benefits for immune function, avoiding infection, reducing cancer risk, etc., and others not clearly showing this benefit. People at risk include those who spend a lot of time indoors and those with darker complexions (harder to absorb). Take with food for better absorption.

Some others that most labs easily measure include folic acid (few are deficient in this, but it's important in pregnancy to reduce neural tube defects).

The Long Supplement List!?

Some of my patients come in with a long list of supplements that they take. I ask them how they decided to take each of the pills. They often relate a magazine or online article they read that suggested a benefit. Sometimes they can't recall what the benefit was supposed to be. When I ask if the article said how long to take the supplement or how to determine a lack of ongoing need for it, most patients are stymied.

So I set a goal of reducing the long list to a shorter list, ideally one-half of the list. This is a starting goal—ultimately we can reduce the list even further. The benefits include financial savings which can be substantial, and a return to a more logical, scientifically based approach to nutrients and supplements.

When you evaluate your supplements, ask:

- Why am I taking this?
- What is the proven benefit?
- How long should I take it?
- How often is appropriate?
- Can I track if it's working?

Also, many supplements have schedules designed by the marketing team, it appears, rather than the health team. So I often advise a B complex to be taken once or twice a week, not daily. Recent research, including the COSMOS trial, suggests multivitamins may have modest cognitive benefits in older adults, though results are still emerging. If you are younger, I don't generally recommend a multivitamin. If you insist, perhaps every other day or twice a week.

Targeted Supplements

I like the idea of targeted supplements. For example, if you take a statin medication for cholesterol or heart issues, some evidence suggests taking CoQ10 may help reduce muscle-related side effects. I typically recommend it about three times a week. Emerging research, including data from the Rotterdam Study, suggests Vitamin K2 may help reduce calcium deposition in arteries, though this remains an area of active investigation.

Eyes

If you have early macular degeneration or a family history of the same, your eye doctor or I may suggest some lutein and zeaxanthin (comes together). This supplement is the key part of the well-documented AREDS2 formula, proven in large National Eye Institute studies to reduce progression of macular degeneration and is likely safe for others and may be protective of vision as we age. Two to three times a week may be sufficient.

Obviously I target whatever is determined on lab testing to be low. If you have a Vitamin D3 below 30, 2000 units a day of D3 for 6–12 months, with a remeasurement, will usually get you to between 35 and 45, a healthy level. If your level is below 20, I'll typically recommend 5000 units D3 a day for 6–12 months with a remeasurement with the goal of 35–45 range. Even a level of 65 is a healthy range for D3, but there is less data on benefit at that level.

Vitamin B12 Levels

Vitamin B12, in healthy people, is usually 450–750. If yours is below 300, I supplement; I don't wait until the 150 or 200 cutoff. Again, monitor with measurements because I have seen a lot of patients who supplement this vitamin go well above 1000 and this is likely not a healthy thing to do. One simply stops taking it for a good while if levels are too high and measures it in 6–12 months.

Supplements can be helpful—but only when they're used thoughtfully, based on your health needs, lab testing, and evidence. A handful of targeted supplements may do more for you than a shelf full of mystery capsules. When in doubt, talk with your doctor about what's worth taking—and what's just making your urine yellow and expensive!

> **Doctor's Note:** *Get your nutrients from food first. Use supplements to fill in gaps, not to build the whole foundation. Focus on supplements with evidence behind their usage.*

SECTION 4

Common Symptoms and Conditions, Part One

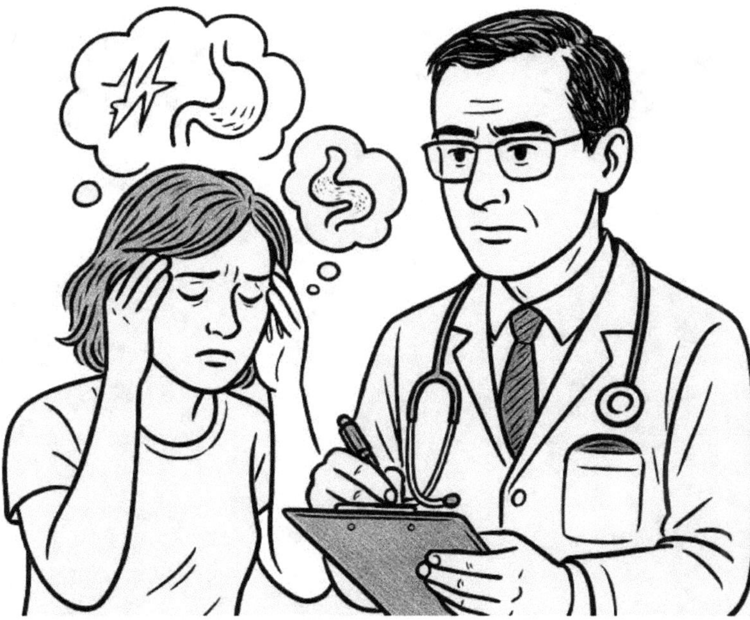

CHAPTER 13

CHRONIC PAIN

I have written books on this subject, including *Think Away Your Pain,* please see the Bibliography. So this section will be dramatically abbreviated, and for those for whom this section resonates, there are books, videos, online courses, and other materials you can learn more from (www.mindbodymedicine.com).

Types of Pain

Some pain is structural, biomechanical, or biochemical in origin. Structural is most common in the acute setting—a sprained ankle that swells up, a fractured wrist, a bruised tailbone after a fall. Biochemically based pain is more common in someone with a rheumatological disease like rheumatoid arthritis, lupus, gout, and the like, which can be detected and diagnosed with detailed blood testing. Biomechanical pain is more common in athletes and as we age. The latter group includes osteoarthritis of the hip or knee. The former group includes a tennis player with poor technique and a sore shoulder or a runner with poor feet or worn out shoes and patellar tendon pain.

Some of the pain I've described above is acute, which typically means in the first six weeks after onset. Some of the above is chronic (more than three or six months) such as osteoarthritis or rheumatoid arthritis. Some of it is subacute (six weeks to three or six months) such as an inflamed shoulder from overuse or a knee injury.

Chronic Pain

Chronic pain is often, however, quite different in nature. This is understood from clinical experience, research, and functional MRI imaging studies. Clinically, patients with chronic pain often don't respond or briefly respond to the types of treatments that help or fix acute pain or injuries. For example, physical therapy, chiropractic, and massage/bodywork. Research shows that a lot of acute pain resolves regardless of what treatment is utilized (Malmivaara and other studies). However, chronic pain can be quite resistant to treatments.

Functional MRI imaging, which I detail in my book in the Chronification chapter, illustrates that the part of the brain that "lights up" with acute pain is the somatosensory cortex. However, in pain that persists more than six months, different parts of the brain are active. Signals are more prominent in the prefrontal cortex, amygdala, and elsewhere, areas that are connected to our emotional centers, as well. So acute pain is a sensory experience. Chronic pain is a nervous system process, a neural circuit condition, (neuroplastic) that is connected to our fears, worries; our psychology, and emotions. Research using functional MRI imaging shows that chronic pain creates actual changes in brain structure and function, which explains why it often doesn't respond to the same treatments that help acute injuries.

Although I learned about this from a mentor, John Sarno M.D., before the availability of functional MRI imaging and other research tools, modern neuroscience matches well and confirms what I learned and practiced. Having this scientific data makes it more real for patients and easier to explain that pain is really "in the brain" and nervous system. It could be said to be in "your head", but not imaginary—just that the brain is the core of the nervous system and that is in your head.

Personality factors can be important in the development and the recovery from chronic pain. Individuals often are highly self-critical, people-pleasers, highly responsible for others, and perfectionists. This generates a great deal of psychological pressure which manifests itself in physical symptoms.

Emotional issues from childhood, teen years, or adulthood are often crucial to understanding and relieving chronic pain. Anger about these traumas is often prominent, although for some, anxiety, fear and grief are equally if not more important. Pain happens to people, not just to the back or the pelvis. Understanding and treating chronic pain involves exploring the totality of a person, not just examining the spine. Unfortunately, the medical profession is often lacking in this biopsychosocial approach.

Neuroplastic Recovery Program

If your chronic pain is diagnosed as neuroplastic or brain-based, there is an effective treatment strategy that includes the correct diagnosis, education via books, video, etc., psychological processing from expressive writing or journaling and sometimes psychotherapy as well. Multiple research studies have shown this approach to be more effective than any other approach including injections or simple cognitive-behavioral therapy (CBT) for chronic pain.

So the correct diagnosis leads to a sometimes unexpected, but usually effective, approach that does require patient acceptance and buy-in to the process. This is not passive treatment like a massage. This is about empowering and guiding a patient to get well and to heal from chronic pain.

Again, appropriate testing to exclude a serious condition and imaging where appropriate is part of the initial workup, or may have already been done before I diagnose a patient with neuroplastic pain or TMS (tension myoneural syndrome).

> ***Doctor's Note:*** *Pain can have physical and emotional roots. Understand and treat the whole person, not just the sore spot.*

CHAPTER 14

UNEXPLAINED SYMPTOMS

Unexplained symptoms are challenging to experience, and obviously, since they are not explained, difficult for the clinicians involved, as well.

Assessment

The first step is to go back to the onset of the problem and really assess where the patient was at that point, physically and emotionally. A careful history focusing on the bio-psycho-social approach pioneered by George Engel, M.D., at Rochester Medical Center 50 years ago is important.

A detailed review of imaging, lab tests, and ordering what needs to be evaluated is also appropriate. There are new cancer screening tests that have become available and no shortage of lab tests or imaging to do.

If nothing shows up, reassurance and support are essential. Validating the symptom as a real sensation, while at the same time staying open to a psychological trigger or precipitant, is crucial. A patient needs to know that the doctor is there for them, even if he/she does not have a clear explanation.

Treatment

How do I treat this? Very similar to chronic pain, above, that is diagnosed as TMS or neuroplastic pain. One can say neuroplastic symptoms if these unexplained symptoms are found to have a pattern indicative of stress, fear, and worry as triggers. If they are inconsistent in when they occur or if they have a peculiar timing (e.g. every night at 9 p.m. or only first thing in the morning).

One continues to see the patient, and where appropriate, specialists, subspecialists, and repeat or other testing can be done if there remains concern about a serious medical condition. But I do focus on getting to understand the patient's life, stressors, past psychological history, traumas, and the like. Often a deeper exploration in this area is more productive than testing ad infinitum. It does require a patient willing to be open to a different explanation for their symptoms and letting go of the connection to a cause such as a vaccine reaction or other connection without clear medical support or evidence.

Also see total body imaging and Galleri MCED testing in the preventive and cancer screening sections.

> ***Doctor's Note:*** *Unexplained doesn't mean imaginary. It's important that your symptoms are validated, that your doctor keeps searching thoughtfully, and stay open to mind-body insights. What you believe about your condition may need to change for your condition to resolve.*

CHAPTER 15

HEADACHES

Headaches are one of mankind's most ubiquitous issues. There are a number of types of headaches. The only ones that are true emergencies are vascular events eliciting headache as a symptom. While rare, they do occur and include ruptured or leaking aneurysm (blood vessel that is enlarged), subdural or epidural hematoma (blood collection in and around the brain that compresses), brain tumors (growths in the skull or brain), and clots in the brain. The telltale sign of these is the "worst headache of your life", a stiff neck, an antecedent fall or trauma, sudden onset of headache ("thunderclap"), or associated changes in mental status or function (vision, speech, movement). Again, these are rare, but important to recognize and go to an emergency room or see a physician immediately.

Most headaches statistically are tension headaches. The pain is from tension in the muscles of the skull, face, or upper neck area that causes, by mechanical traction or other means, sensory signals and pain. These headaches can be mild or severe, last hours or rarely days or longer, but are not dangerous. Diagnosis includes excluding other types of headache by examination (neurologic testing) and sometimes imaging (CT or MRI scan). Treatment could be as simple as a hot shower, hot towel, ice pack, gentle massage, or stretching. Psychological tension can feed into the muscles and this can be a mind-body disorder. Medications including NSAIDs (Advil/Aleve), acetaminophen (Tylenol), or muscle relaxants (cyclobenzaprine, methocarbamol) can help relieve symptoms or break the cycle of pain.

Mixed-tension-vascular headaches have elements of tension headache, but also elements of a vascular syndrome. The classic vascular headache is called a migraine and may have a classic aura or warning symptoms which might include flashing lights, visual field issues, etc. The migraine is usually a one-sided (unilateral) headache and may localize behind an eye, or in the forehead or side of the head. A mixed tension-vascular headache may have some, but not all, of these features and also a tension element.

Classic Migraine

The classic migraine can be brought on by loud noise, bright lights, stress, smells, etc. There are effective medications like sumatriptan (and other triptans) which can be taken orally, sublingual (under the tongue), nasal spray, or injectable to quickly abort the headache or break the cycle. Sometimes, a quiet room, slow breathing, and relaxing can help. Migraines seem to run in families, suggesting a genetic element, but stress, emotional tension, and worry can also be a significant factor.

Cluster Headache

Another headache which is severe and usually affects men is the cluster headache. This is often described as a knife-like pain through one eye and may involve testing of the eye and other symptoms. Sometimes breathing pure oxygen can help, and there are medications that can break a seasonal cycle of cluster headaches, which some individuals get. Intravenous medications are sometimes used in severe cases, and prednisone or the equivalent is one of the medications that helps to break the cycle.

For most people with a new onset of headaches, a careful exam by a family doctor or neurologist is necessary and imaging, ideally MRI. If there are no structural issues, the treatments mentioned above can help a lot. Posture, computer use, phone use, and stress should all be evaluated—Headaches can be related to lots of emotional factors (see prior sections on mind-body issues.) Once we clarify the type of headache through your symptoms, history, and examination, treatment becomes more focused and effective—and many headache cycles can be broken.

Doctor's Note: *Most headaches aren't dangerous, but they can be debilitating. Identify triggers, recognize patterns, and know the difference between tension, migraine, and emergency. The right diagnosis leads to the right treatment—and relief.*

CHAPTER 16

Joint Issues

Let's speak generally and then more specifically about the joints in your body.

First, what are the joints? They are areas of our skeleton that can bend and twist. As you know, the center of a bone won't bend or twist unless it is broken! However, elbows, knees, ankles, and wrists, to mention several joints, do have the capacity to bend, twist, and sometimes rotate as well to allow us more sophisticated types of movements.

What can happen to joints? Like most of our body, we take our joints for granted when they are working well. However, when they hurt or are stiff, we really notice the difference. Acute problems with our joints (of recent origin) would be injuries, sprains, other inflammation, aches, and pains. Chronic issues with our joints include arthritis, arthralgias (pain, not inflamed), tendon and ligament issues, and cartilage problems.

Let's go through these a bit.

Knees

Knees are perhaps the joint I see most often with pain or functional limitations. I start with the history of the problem. A knee problem for five years is different from a knee problem for a week. A knee problem that affects your tennis is different from a knee problem that stops you from walking a flight of stairs.

Examination is very helpful for the knees. I start off by asking the patient to stand and then squat. If they can do this adequately, I have them repeat it. Someone who can squat and arise twice without pain almost always does not have a meniscus tear. A meniscus tear is a piece of cushioning cartilage that is ripped. Sometimes it requires surgery, and other times rehabilitation can allow enough healing to allow you to return to your activities. Healing a meniscus is challenging, because its blood supply is limited and it gets nutrients from joint fluid. Not a recipe for fast healing, at all. In contrast, your scalp and face have abundant blood supply, as do your bones!

Many of the knee issues I see fall into pain from mechanical dysfunction in or near the patella or kneecap. These are treated with exercises including strengthening of the quads (thigh muscles) and hamstrings, the glutes (buttocks muscles) and stretching of these associated areas. Riding a stationary bicycle is a clear winner when it comes to rehabilitating the knee. The bike removes a lot of the weight-bearing pain and allows good range of motion of the knee (although not full) and strengthening of the quads. Swimming can also be helpful as a rehab device, as can running in shallow water (depth of water determines the buoyancy you get and hence the reduction in weight forces on the knee. Speaking of weight, a long-term benefit for the knees is to reduce any excess weight down to a normal or ideal range.

Arthritic Knees

Another set of knee issues I see falls into the medical diagnosis of osteoarthritis. Arthritis is inflammation of a joint (arth is joint, -itis is inflammation); it is wear and tear of the articular (joint covering) cartilage and a reduction in the smooth gliding in comparison to a healthy joint. The articular cartilage is different from meniscus cartilage in location and in physical properties. For arthritic knees, I typically see pain with squatting, sometimes painful and reduced range of motion, and sometimes localized tenderness as well. X-rays are the best diagnostic test for osteoarthritis. Osteoarthritis is associated with aging and has genetic elements as well. For some individuals, cumulative wear and tear causes osteoarthritic changes. But this does not mean we should spend our lives lying down to avoid OA. This has its own set of complications. Stay active.

Cross-train if you get into your thirties or forties (or fifties) and begin to find that daily running or four times a week tennis is too much for your knees (or other joints). Cross-training means varying your activities. An example of a cross-training week might be Monday jogging, Tuesday swimming, Wednesday tennis, Thursday biking, Friday jog or swim, Saturday yoga. You could also mix in weight training with 2 or more of those exercise days. Weight training, strength training, or resistance training is spoken of in similar terms. So actual free weights, machines, elastic bands, or body weight push-ups, pull-ups, and planks can function as great strength and resistance exercises.

Often patients with mild to moderate osteoarthritis get a great deal of improvement in pain and function with cross-training and modifying activities. In addition, icing the knee (or other joint) can be very helpful. An ice pack for 5–10 minutes is typically adequate. On the subject of ice, the closer to the surface a structure is, the shorter the interval of icing needed to cool down the area. No area should be iced for more than 20 minutes due to risk of injury to adjacent nerves and soft tissues. If discomfort is too severe, obviously remove the ice or ice pack. I like ice packs, but a bag of frozen peas or corn in a ziplock bag is great for the smaller joints (wrist, ankle, etc.) because this conforms to the shape of the joint and typically retains that shape when you refreeze it. Also, there is no accumulation of water, like with actual ice, as it melts.

Advanced Treatments for Joints

There are, of course, treatments beyond the above for joint problems. I mentioned imaging with x-rays is typically the first level of this. Injections are another set of options. The most common injection involves a cortisone derivative like triamcinolone (Kenalog) or the equivalent. People ask about risks. Repeated injections (more than three in a year) to the same joint are typically unwise. However, in decades of injecting joints, I have seen very few, and minor, negative effects of injections. Cortisone is more risky to the entire body when taken orally or used for a longer period of time. Another type of injection I find beneficial is hyaluronic acid (Hylagan, Synvisc, etc.). This is similar to a lubricant injected into the joint that lasts for months and often provides immediate benefit (even as the patient walks off the injection table and goes to the front desk!). I have found this to be safe and well tolerated in the hands of a physician with experience and skills in accurate positioning of the injections.

Beyond these two, are PRP and stem cells. This is an evolving area, and I discuss risks, benefits, and alternatives carefully with patients. PRP is platelet-rich plasma. The process is to typically draw your blood and put it through a special centrifuge process to remove much of the serum (liquid) and red blood cells while retaining platelets (little clotting cells), some plasma, and perhaps some white cells and other components related to healing. An analogy would be the cells and fluids that come into a cut to, seemingly miraculously, heal the cut. In nature this requires no effort at all. In medicine, the process is more time consuming and hence more expensive. (Five times as expensive in comparison to above injections, or more.)

More costly than this is stem cell injection. While there are a number of ways to obtain stem cells, including umbilical cord blood, most commonly it is extracted from your fat cells in the outside of your abdomen, purified and then injected into the joint. This process is more complicated and more expensive (5x to PRP). I would only consider PRP and stem cells for a patient who has done everything else and whose options are starting to lean toward knee replacement surgery.

Other Joints

There are a lot of other joints, and I will mention some specific issues for them while not going into as many details as I have done with knees. There are many similarities in treatment for each of our joints, and some differences.

Hips

For hips, another common area for osteoarthritis (and less common for other forms of arthritis), injections are more complicated due to the depth one must inject to get the medication into the joint. I have typically referred this to a radiologist who can do it under X-ray guidance. Some doctors do it with ultrasound guidance and others by anatomic landmarks alone. On the other hand, when the hip has gotten very restricted in range of motion and the x-rays confirm severe osteoarthritis, I am not hesitant to refer my patients for total hip replacement. This surgery has become very successful for a high percentage of hip arthritis sufferers. Recovery is surprisingly quick, and I have patients hiking, playing pickleball, walking five miles regularly, and doing other activities after hip replacement. The one activity not advised is running due to the wear and tear this activity can produce on the hip. Each step in a jog may cause 3-5x our weight to be transmitted to our hips. Walking is more like 1.5 to 2x.

Shoulders

For shoulders, perhaps the most complicated joints we have, injections and physical therapy are the mainstays. Surgery is appropriate for a smaller number of individuals, and joint replacement is still in the more primitive stages of technical advancement. It is a complicated joint because our shoulder is designed for us to move in all the directions of the compass—and more. Probably we evolved to throw rocks at our prey (and our enemies), as well as reach, pull, and lift and hence the joint is designed to be less stable but more flexible than any other major joint. Rehabilitation is complicated, so I advise physical therapy rather than home exercises for almost anyone with shoulder tendinitis, minor rotator cuff tear, or other condition of the shoulder. As noted, injections can dramatically reduce inflammation and pain and allow adherence to exercise and PT.

One troubling condition of the shoulder I will mention is frozen shoulder (aka adhesive capsulitis). This typically develops in individuals 40–60 years old and is somewhat more common in women. In Chinese medicine books from two thousand years ago, they called it the fifty-year-old shoulder! Despite being known about for millennia, our understanding of this condition is still not complete, and our treatment approaches are frankly quite limited. I have had this condition myself (sequentially, in both shoulders), so I know a lot about the condition from reading, taking care of patients, and personal experience.

The diagnosis can be difficult as early stages appear identical to tendonitis (inflammation of a tendon) or impingement syndrome (tendon irritation due to reduced space) of the shoulder. At some point, the patient, or the doctor, notices a dramatically reduced range of motion of the shoulder. Here's a special point. In most tendinitis and rotator cuff syndrome, the shoulder can be passively moved by the examiner. This is where the patient relaxes and the doctor or therapist moves the shoulder through an arc of motion. In frozen shoulders, this does not succeed. The joint is frozen and it won't move regardless of patient effort or lack of effort.

The stages of frozen shoulder have classically been described as freezing (weeks to months), frozen (months), and thawing (months). During phase 1 and early phase 2, several studies have suggested that cortisone injections into the glenohumeral (shoulder) joint may shorten the phases slightly or considerably. So I do try to provide these injections during the first few months. They are not believed to be effective after that. The typical shoulder injection is subacromial, so this injection is done a little deeper and at a slightly different location. Ultrasound guidance or experience can help make this an accurate one. Physical therapy can play a role in all stages to reduce discomfort, encourage movement, and eventually to speed thawing. I do not find that some of the scary lengths (1–2 years) described in some articles on this condition are accurate. For most patients, 3–9 months leads to complete resolution, hopefully on the shorter end of this range. MRI imaging may show typical findings of a pouch or tightened joint that shows the pathologic process of severe joint inflammation and fibrosis in this condition. Again, fortunately, it typically resolves with minimal or no residual limitations.

Ankles

Ankles are another area that is a common sports injury and can also occur with a fall or minor accident. Ankles seem to respond well to the RICE model of therapy.—Rest, ice, compression, elevation. Add gentle range of motion as tolerated, ankle bracing in the acute phase, and avoid premature return to basketball or other ankle-dangerous sports (volleyball, tennis, etc.) They do heal, although once you've sprained an ankle twice, it does seem more vulnerable to respraining. One element of rehabilitation or PT that is very important for ankles is proprioception. This describes one's ability to sense our position in space. This can be damaged in the ankle along with the soft tissue sprain, swelling, and pain. A balance board is the best way to retrain our ankles for the proprioception needed for basketball, dancing, and other agility sports and activities. Functional ankle bracing, worn under the shoe, can be helpful when one returns to sports. The ankle walker, or boot, is used in the acute phase of severe sprains (and even minor fractures), to allow limited walking in a restricted boot, and the support one needs to move around without pain, and usually without crutches.

Wrists

Wrists can be injured, and assuming no fracture to the two rows of wrist bones, with the scaphoid being the most hazardous bone to break, usually bracing and time are quite effective to help healing.

Some chronic wrist issues respond to a cortisone injection. A not uncommon issue in women breastfeeding their first infant and in some other individuals with wrist movements in uncomfortable positions is an easily diagnosable and treatable condition called De Quervain's tenosynovitis (like tendonitis). De Quervain's has a specific finding on the exam, and once I diagnose it, I advise a shot. The injection is with a small needle, and a small amount of cortisone mixed with lidocaine is remarkably well tolerated, safe, easy, and effective. PT and other alternatives take longer, and especially for a woman who is lactating, time with the baby and without pain is of the essence.

Elbows

Elbows are less likely to be inflamed in the joint itself although we see a lot of epicondylitis (inflammation of the inner or outer soft tissue adjacent to the elbow). The term tennis elbow or golf elbow is the lay term for this condition. Treatment may include modifying tennis grip or technique, ice, local creams, or less commonly injection. The topical I advise for this condition and for joints in general, where we like to avoid oral medications if we can, is diclofenac (or Voltaren) gel. This is over the counter in the US for ten years and in Europe and elsewhere for much longer. So it is safe for most people and well tolerated and effective for musculoskeletal conditions, especially those that are close to the surface. Think of the equivalent of Advil/Aleve, but rubbed on the area injured.

> **Doctor's Note:** *Joints bear the weight of our active lives. Stay ahead of problems with cross-training, proper form, and early intervention. Most joint issues respond well to conservative care—but don't wait too long to address persistent pain.*

CHAPTER 17

DIGESTIVE HEALTH

As a family doctor, I see a lot of patients with concerns about digestion, bloating, acid reflux, abdominal pain, and diarrhea. As it is for other areas of health, one of my roles is to determine who needs to see a sub-specialist, a gastroenterologist.

For the acute gastro issues, I see food poisoning and gastroenteritis. The former hits quickly and resolves fairly quickly. More likely to have vomiting as well as diarrhea, and people can sometimes describe other members of their family or dining party who also became ill. Viral gastroenteritis is actually more common. The challenge for patients (and their doctors) is that we eat three times a day, most of us, so there is always a meal or a food item to blame if we feel an upset stomach or diarrhea. But usually it turns out to be a viral infection rather than bad food that is the cause.

The good news is that many acute gastro issues are self-limiting and resolve or improve dramatically within three days on their own. I talk to patients about hydration if they are having diarrhea or vomiting. We discuss a BRAT diet (bananas, rice, apples(-auce), toast, and tea), and in cases of nausea, a great prescription medication called ondansetron (or Zofran) which can rapidly control nausea in most people. It even comes in an orally dissolving tablet, so if nauseated, you don't have to swallow the pill!

Pepto-bismol may be helpful or kaopectate for diarrhea. Both are taken orally as liquid over the counter medication.

Chronic GI Issues

For more chronic GI distress, I ask about symptoms, and may suggest fiber or probiotics or both. Fiber is great for constipation and may help with chronic loose stools as well. My favorite is methylcellulose (Citrucel) but psyllium husk (Metamucil) is also an excellent choice. One to two Citrucel tablets a day can take someone who is chronically constipated and give them a more regular bowel pattern. The tablet version is easier to consume than the historically known powder in eight ounces of water. For people with gas and bloating, this may also help a lot. I give the analogy of a train that arrives a day late at the station. Annoying. Same thing if the bowel movement you should have had last night you get today. Fiber may improve the timing and regularity and therefore reduce the accumulation or passage of intestinal gas.

Probiotics, either in capsule/tablet form, or in food form as a fermented food (yogurt, kimchi, sauerkraut), may allow our microbiome (the bacteria that normally reside in the colon) to regulate and become a better balance for us. The challenge is that it is hard to determine if you have a bacterial insufficiency, a bacterial overgrowth, or the wrong combination of bacteria. So a bit of trial and error at this point. Testing that claims to tell us what the patient needs in the gut has not proven useful, in my experience.

Abdominal Pain

Appendicitis generally manifests with acute right lower abdominal pain and tenderness on exam. There are other findings on examination, as well. An emergency room and a CT scan usually follow, along with a surgical consult. It is rare to see this in outpatient practice, more so in urgent care or emergency rooms.

Right upper quadrant pain episodes, possibly with a physical exam finding called a Murphy's sign, are more common. For this, I obtain an abdominal ultrasound to confirm the presence of gallstones. Some people need surgical referral and consideration for removal of the gallbladder. Others modify their diet, with less fatty food, and monitor their symptoms closely over time, doing well. Gallstones can also be asymptomatic and picked up incidentally. At this time, recommendations are to observe these patients rather than intervene. Medications to dissolve gallstones have not proven consistently successful at this time.

Acid Reflux

Acid reflux, or gastroesophageal reflux (GERD), is a common and annoying condition. Initially I advise some simple measures that may help. Both over-the-counter, like calcium carbonate (e.g. TUMS) or magnesium hydroxide (e.g. Maalox) and prescription medications can also resolve symptoms. We start with eating meals earlier in the evening, NOT lying down after eating, instead sitting or standing/walking, and sometimes elevating one's head while sleeping. Alcohol can be a trigger as can acidic foods like tomato sauce. Smaller, more frequent meals and chewing one's food very completely may also help.

Adding occasional famotidine (Pepcid) for flare ups may help mild cases and daily famotidine for more moderate cases may control symptoms. Another OTC option is omeprazole (Prilosec). For more severe and recurrent reflux symptoms, I may prescribe pantoprazole (Protonix) which is taken a half hour before dinner or breakfast or both, and helps a lot, but people may become dependent on it. It's easier to go on Protonix than get off of it in my experience, but it is also effective in treatment. For more severe symptoms, especially those that persist, a gastroenterologist referral with a likely upper GI endoscopy (scope that looks down the throat to the stomach) is important to ensure the diagnosis is correct and there is nothing worrisome.

Doctor's Note: *Most digestive issues are manageable with simple interventions—fiber, probiotics, dietary changes. But persistent symptoms deserve attention. Learn when to try home remedies and when to seek medical evaluation.*

CHAPTER 18

THE UPPER RESPIRATORY INFECTION: COLDS AND FLU

This was easy before Covid-19 in 2020. Most upper respiratory infections (URIs) were caused by viruses associated with the common cold. Treatment was supportive, and people got better in three to ten days, with seven to ten days being common. People were contagious early on, and good hand-washing, avoiding coughing and sneezing in people's faces, and washing items at home kept other people relatively safe. Children get more colds than adults, and some people innately have great resistance to getting sick with the "common cold". Some people get 3–5 colds a year and that is normal for them.

Obviously, our experience with Covid-19 has changed us all. This pandemic came in with a bang, initially produced dramatically sick people, in many cases, and led to shutdowns, isolation, and other public health-derived restrictions. So that was a few years ago and as of this writing, Covid is a milder illness, rarely causing hospitalization or serious illness. The biggest risk is to an elderly, debilitated person. A combination of natural immunity, vaccine-derived immunity, and viral mutation has brought us to this current stage of being aware of Covid, but not obsessed by it.

Home Treatment

So what do you do if you develop upper respiratory symptoms? One thing we've learned is that it is better to stay at home and work from home, if you can, and partially isolate yourself to reduce the spread of the virus you are harboring. The Japanese did this well before Covid-19. They usually mask when ill and try to keep others safe. Their culture mandates this type of concern and you saw Japanese people in airports with masks before Covid hit and wondered, why? Now we know.

Fluids, acetaminophen, rest, and other over-the-counter remedies are the primary focus for management of upper respiratory infections. An exception is a severe sore throat, often with fever, usually without cough. For this, a strep test can be done, usually a rapid one, in the office. If strep is detected, patients improve faster with antibiotics, and the rare risk of a strep complication is averted. Otherwise, most URIs are viruses, and most are the common cold.

Flu

During flu season, which varies, but December through March is an approximate estimate, depending on your geographic location, if you get an illness with high fever and muscle aches, headache, getting checked for flu with a rapid flu test can lead to a prescription for Tamiflu (oseltamivir)—or equivalent. This is an antiviral medication specifically treating Influenza A. It often reduces the severity or duration of illness, but perhaps by a day or so. I prescribed it regularly before Covid-19. Interestingly, during Covid, with all the masking, working from home, and distancing, there was a year or two where almost no one got the flu! Masking didn't stop Covid from spreading, but it did stop the flu! In fact, the quadrivalent flu shot (four strains) was changed to a trivalent shot this year (2024–5) because one of the strains had vanished! Apparently this was a natural shift from that period of Covid.

Covid

So what if you test at home, or at the doctor's office or clinic, and you have Covid. First, don't panic. Second, put on a mask to keep others safe. Third, go home and rest, drink fluids, take acetaminophen, and use other over-the-counter supportive medications. Most people ride it out like a cold or a flu and return to work in about five days, or after symptoms have resolved. How about Paxlovid? Individual decision, but this is a medication with drug interactions, potential side effects and not amazing effectiveness. Hence I rarely prescribe it. It's primarily used in vulnerable populations early in the illness to reduce the risk of severe disease. Fortunately, for most people, this year, the risk of severe disease is very, very low.

What about the myriad of over-the-counter options. Again, acetaminophen is a favorite. Ibuprofen or naproxen are also excellent. If fever is high, you can even overlap these medications. By that I mean take acetaminophen at noon. You can't repeat it until 6 or 8 p.m. depending on dosage. But if fever persists at 3 or 4 p.m., you can take ibuprofen safely and then take acetaminophen at 8 p.m.. Maximum daily acetaminophen dosage for short periods is 3000 mg (e.g. three of the 1000 mg tablets or 4 of the 750 mg in a day). Longer-term, the less medication, the better.

Cough Medications

Dextromethorphan (DM) has a mild anti-cough benefit. Tessalon Perles, which is prescribed, also has anti-tussive (cough-reducing) properties and helps some folks. I am a big fan of breathing steam, in the shower, from boiling water, or another device, to help irritated mucous membranes in the nose and bronchial tree. Tea is also a fine option. Chicken soup has some of the same heat, steam properties, and may have other antiviral benefits as well! Vicks Vaporub (menthol and other ingredients), which has been around forever, also has some benefits on cough, confirmed in research studies!

Guaifenesin (like Robitussin-DM and others) is also used for cough and has mild benefits on thinning mucus and is called an expectorant. The goal is to thin phlegm and bring it up, either cough it out, or swallow it, rather than have it remain inside the body to annoy us and block our passages.

Nasal sprays were touched on before, but oxymetazoline (Afrin) has some nasal stuffiness benefits and works quickly. One must avoid using it for longer than three to four days due to a rebound effect where you get worse without realizing it's the medication not the illness.

Speaking of getting worse, if you have a cold for 5–7 days and then get worse, that's when your doctor may be of help. It could be a sinus infection (sinusitis), which can manifest with yellow-green or neon nasal mucous discharge. You might have pneumonia, if your lungs are more congested and you feel short of breath or are producing thick sputum when you cough. Finally, if you have asthma, a worsening might indicate bronchospasm and the need for your inhalers or to see the doctor to get additional oral medications or other inhaled medication.

Vitamins?

Does Vitamin C help? Some people believe it does, but the evidence is not really there. If you believe it will help, however, there may be a benefit from a placebo response. Does echinacea work? The evidence is not really there, same comment.

Zinc lozenges may help with sore throats or colds in the early stages. Multiple studies have supported some benefit in reducing symptoms and shortening the duration of the illness. These lozenges dissolve under the tongue and taste okay. Try them early on. Follow package directions.

Does Vitamin D help? There was some initial interest in this for Covid. Taking some can't hurt you. Many people are Vitamin D deficient, but if you are not, it probably won't make much difference. Another reasonable "placebo" choice for your upper respiratory infection or Covid.

Antibiotics

Antibiotics? Great if you have a bacterial infection. However, most URIs are viral. When can this help you? An acute sinus infection (see above). Pneumonia can be bacterial, although not always. An ear infection. Strep throat. Persistent bronchitis may be bacterial. So that is why your doctor won't prescribe a "z-pak". The overuse of antibiotics in the US and elsewhere has led to the development of bacteria that are resistant to the antibiotics we have. This is a problem. This problem can be minimized or stopped from worsening if we only use antibiotics when absolutely necessary. Otherwise, they won't work when we really need them.

Fluids, rest, acetaminophen, tea, and steam are the go-tos in my life and my practice for colds and flus. The body has an amazing ability to recover, give it rest, fluids, and time, and it usually does a great job. We are impatient creatures and, of course, want a quick fix. Sometimes there is none, and that is hard to accept in the modern world.

> **Doctor's Note:** *Most colds and flu just need time, fluids, and rest. Your immune system does the heavy lifting. Antibiotics don't help viruses. Know the warning signs of complications, but trust your body to heal most upper respiratory infections on its own.*

SECTION 5

Common Symptoms and Conditions, Part Two

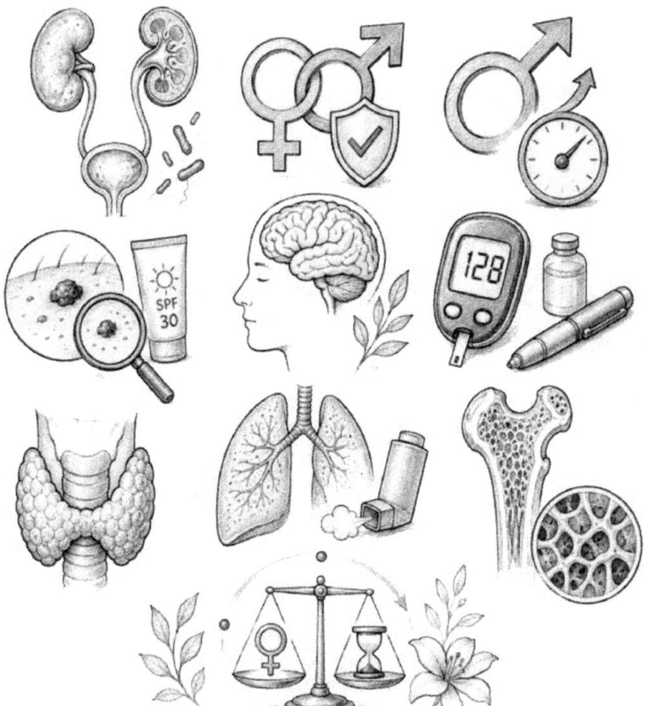

CHAPTER 19
URINARY TRACT INFECTIONS

Urinary tract infections (UTI's) are only peripherally related to sexually transmitted infections... in some cases. By this I mean that in some sexually active women, intercourse may lead to a UTI. The example of "honeymoon cystitis" is when a woman, either not sexually active, or infrequently active, spends a lot of time with her partner, has more sex than usual, and gets a UTI. Some women find it helpful to urinate after sex to reduce risks of UTI's. Staying hydrated is also important

UTI's happen in men, as well, but they are less common in younger, healthy men and more common in aging men. Some of these infections can be quite serious in the elderly and even lead to sepsis or a blood infection where the urinary bacteria spread in the circulatory system. This must be aggressively treated if it occurs. Healthy men can get UTI's and the thinking is that if it happens twice, further workup of the bladder and kidneys is appropriate. For women, workup is not advised for simple UTI's of the bladder, but recurrent kidney infections (pyelonephritis) may necessitate further testing.

Treatment

Ideally, a urine specimen is obtained and a portion of this midstream, clean catch specimen is sent for a culture. Treatment can begin before the culture results are back; they take 2–4 days and may include bacterial sensitivity testing which is helpful for being specific about treatment, especially if response is slow.

A urine analysis, either by dipstick or microscopic, can reveal lots of white cells in a patient suffering from a UTI. Bacteria may also be seen in abundance, and sometimes some red cells, as well.

Empiric treatment is based upon allergies and symptoms. For cystitis (bladder only infection), the amoxicillin family, sulfa antibiotics like trimethoprim/sulfamethoxazole (bactrim DS) or nitrofurantoin (macrodantin) or cephalosporins like cephalexin (keflex) are good choices.

I try to avoid ciprofloxacin (cipro), which can often be effective. I also strongly avoid levofloxacin (levaquin). Why? Both of these antibiotics have been associated with an increased likelihood of tendon rupture and related musculoskeletal injuries (tendonitis). I prefer to avoid these risks since there are good alternatives to these medications. Some doctors are still too casual with these medications despite black box warnings about this fluoroquinolone category of antibiotics.

Kidney infections may require intravenous or intramuscular medication in some situations.

Doctor's Note: *Urinary tract infections are common, relatively easily diagnosed, and successfully treated. I avoid fluoroquinolone antibiotics because of tendon risks with cipro and levaquin. There are other excellent options. Frequent infections may require further testing.*

CHAPTER 20

SEXUALLY TRANSMITTED ILLNESSES

The terminology here can vary with the acronym STIs or the older STDs. In any event, there should be no stigma. Also, prevention is still the best option.

Prevention

Prevention can be multifactorial. A monogamous relationship with a faithful partner is the lowest risk environment regarding STIs. In a new sexual relationship, or with multiple partners, the use of condoms is an essential barrier element to reduce infection transmission. The "safe sex" option of no exchange of bodily fluids is also an option for some. With new relationships, insisting on both partners being tested before beginning intercourse is a valuable way to reduce exposure to illness.

PREP: Pre Exposure Prophylaxis

For higher risk groups, including MSM (men having sex with men), PREP medication, taken daily, can dramatically reduce the risk of acquiring the AIDS virus. Blood tests are obtained at initiation (HIV and other STIs) and at regular followup visits (typically every 3 months) and a prescription for a medication such as Truvada or Descovy is written. Note that the PREP medication is not an adequate treatment for HIV infection, so HIV testing must be regularly done. It is, however, an option for prevention.

PEP: Post Exposure Prophylaxis

Post exposure medication is given to individuals who may have been exposed to the HIV virus during sexual relations or a needle stick situation. The medication is given for twenty eight days, so it is a much bigger commitment in time and effort. It must be started within 72 hours of exposure; the sooner the better. Up to three medications may be recommended. Side effects are more common.

DOXY-PEP: Post exposure

Doxycycline post exposure prophylaxis is the use of 200mg of doxycycline taken within 72 hours after condomless sex to prevent bacterial sexually transmitted infections Specifically syphilis, chlamydia, and gonorrhea. It is highly effective for men who have sex with men (MSM) and transgender women, reducing risk by roughly two-thirds. Again, condoms and preventive measures are still more effective. This doesn't replace PREP for HIV prevention.

Common STIs.

Gonorrhea is common and in men produces a yellowish green penile discharge in most cases. Chlamydia is even more common and produces a more watery discharge in most men. Both of these conditions may present without symptoms, especially, but not exclusively in women. Testing is mostly by urine sample— amplified DNA is looked for in the specimen.

Syphilis is less common, but potentially very serious. It is mostly detected with blood testing. Unusual rashes may rarely lead to the diagnosis, or even unusual findings on eye exam!

Hepatitis C is detected on blood testing. There is now effective treatment for Hepatitis C, but it involves a long course of medications.

HIV is well known and can be detected with a blood test. Treatment is far more effective than in the past. Many individuals go to undetectable levels of virus with the treatment, which needs to be continued life-long.

All of these tests can be obtained at a doctor's office and sent to a laboratory. Some individuals seek out a clinic to do this testing if they are seeking anonymity or cost savings.

Doctor's Note: *Human beings engage in sexual relations. There should be no stigma associated with asking for prevention or treatment. Start with prevention, where possible, and understand the other options above to reduce risk.*

CHAPTER 21

ERECTILE DYSFUNCTION

Many men suffer from erectile dysfunction (ED) as they age, or in association with vascular conditions or other medical issues. I will also note that the concept of erectile dissatisfaction is another category of men who are getting erections, but not quite what they would like or what they remember. The two categories of men I most commonly see are the younger, sexually active male who gets anxious with a new partner and the medication provides confidence and the older male seeking a rejuvenation of penile function.

Meds for ED

These PDE-5 (phosphodiesterase-5) medications have been available for over twenty five years. They illustrate a key principle because they were initially very expensive (I can recall $50 per pill) and are now generic and very inexpensive (often under 50 cents per pill!). They are effective for most men. Tadalafil (Cialis) is a great option because it can last a few days in one's system or be taken daily in lower dosages. Sildenafil (Viagra) works a bit faster but is typically out of the system in hours or a day. Risks of these meds are an erection that does not go down. If this occurs, one must go to an emergency room for treatment. This is fortunately quite rare.

I prefer to start patients with small to medium dosages; as always in medicine, start low, go slow. One can always increase the dosage, and as inexpensive as these meds have become, the patient can be advised to take a second pill if needed. If too strong, splitting in half is another option, although these pills seem to have always been printed in odd shapes, harder to cut.

In extremely unusual cases, these medications don't work and I may prescribe creams or penile injections, the latter usually with the involvement of a urologist. ED may correlate with cardiovascular disease, especially in younger middle aged men (45–55), where it is less common. ED can be vascular, neurologic, or psychologic in cause. Vascular is more common as we age.

Doctor's Note: *Erectile dysfunction is common as men age and treatment is effective with reasonably safe, inexpensive medication options.*

CHAPTER 22

Skin Health: Understanding Growths, Moles, and Prevention

Skin Bumps: Significant?

Self-assessing your skin isn't just about identifying growths but also fostering a habit of regular monitoring, so that you're aware of changes early on.

In fact, nearly everyone has growths and moles on their skin, especially as they age. How do you know if a growth is something of concern? First of all, see your primary care doctor regularly for checkups or physicals. The doctor can look at any growth and advise you whether to have a dermatologist inspect them. Another option is yearly visits to a dermatologist. This is especially important if you have a personal or family history of melanoma. A personal history of other skin cancers (basal cell, squamous) also necessitates regular dermatology visits for the rest of your life.

But let's say you want to self-assess (not self-diagnose) a skin lesion.

ABCDE Rule

Use the ABCDE Rule. It's very helpful. The letters are obviously alphabetical, but the order is not the order of priorities; it's just a useful mnemonic tied to the first five letters.

A is asymmetrical. A symmetrical lesion (round) is less likely to be a skin cancer than one that includes asymmetric elements. But this is NOT a hard and fast rule.

B is borders. Irregular borders (uneven, like a coastline) can be of concern. Smooth borders are less worrisome. Again, there are exceptions.

C is color. This is a very important factor. Skin-colored and light brown lesions are much less likely to be a cancer than black ones, especially when there are other colors (like blue) mixed in with the black. Pearly white lesions can also be a kind of skin cancer.

D is diameter. Larger is often worse. So something that is larger than a pencil eraser may be of more concern. But there are also small melanomas (dark lesions), so it's not a perfect rule.

E is evolution. This is the most important factor. A changing lesion is far more concerning than something you've had since age fifteen or age five months. Change is the process by which a benign, perhaps congenital (from birth) lesion is transformed (from sun exposure or other factors) into something worrisome that should be examined, perhaps biopsied or removed.

When to Worry

If any of the following apply, it's time to make an appointment with your doctor:

1. You notice any changes in size, shape, or color.
2. A mole bleeds, itches, or feels painful.
3. You've never seen the mole before or it shows up suddenly in an area not previously exposed to the sun.

Types of Skin Lesions

Most skin lesions are benign and these include most freckles, seborrheic keratoses (often have a stuck-on appearance) which are associated with aging and sun exposure, and angiomas (red, blood vessel growths).

The ones we worry about are the pre-cancerous lesions like actinic keratoses. Your dermatologist can find these and remove them. Skin cancers are either basal cell (usually stays local, but can invade adjacent tissue), squamous cell (can be seen on extremities as well), and the worst is melanoma which can spread and can occasionally be fatal. Sores that don't heal, lesions that you scratch and come back, growths that bleed or change in some way are the biggest concerns here.

Skin Biopsy

What is a skin biopsy? Usually it's a removal of the mole in question. Dermatologists and family doctors do a lot of shave excisions to remove lesions from 1 mm up to 10 mm or a little more. Larger lesions may need a different kind of excision, and in those cases, there may be sutures to place and to remove. Shave excisions heal without sutures although they may leave a small scar in the area. Your doctor will decide. In rare cases, skin lesions are partially removed in the biopsy process and the rest is left intact. This might apply to very large lesions or for other reasons.

The tissue that is removed, in any of these cases, will be sent to a lab where a pathologist will examine it under a microscope and render a pathologic diagnosis—hopefully congenital nevus (benign), blue nevus (benign), and rarely basal cell cancer (malignant, but doesn't spread far or have a chance of killing you). The worst diagnosis is, of course, melanoma, which is a more serious kind of skin cancer. Typically the dermatologist will need to do a wider, deeper excision, and depending on local spread and other factors, additional treatments may be required. Early stage melanoma may only require the deep excision and monitoring. More serious cases may need lymph node dissection or chemotherapy. Treatments have improved over the years.

Prevention

Prevention is key. Basic prevention is sunscreen, hats, and appropriate clothing to protect the skin. We've learned that children, especially, who spend more time in the sun than most adults do, need to be protected. Sunscreen would typically be SPF 30+, zinc based is now considered safest. Reapply sunscreen frequently when outside.

Advanced prevention and early detection would include close monitoring of any skin growths with the ABCDE Rule, with preventive medical checkups, and the like. Take ten minutes today and look at yourself in the mirror, and if you have a significant other, ask them to do so as well. Frequency of skin examinations should be individualized based upon family history, number of lesions, current sun exposure, skin and eye color, and childhood or teen cumulative sun exposures.

Keep Checking

The bottom line: keep an eye on your skin and have your family doctor do the same—perhaps involving a dermatologist for higher-risk patients. Prevention matters: use sunscreen, wear hats, and cover up. Sunburns accelerate skin aging and increase cancer risk. Examine your skin regularly at home in good light, including your back with help from a partner or mirror. You may wish to take photos of less visible areas like your back and check them later. Your dermatologist may also do photos as part of her examination.

Doctor's Note: *Your skin tells a story—pay attention to it. Use the ABCDE Rule, protect yourself from sun damage, and get suspicious moles checked early. Skin cancer is highly treatable when caught in time.*

CHAPTER 23

Mental Health and Stress Management

Mental health challenges are varied. Common diagnoses are anxiety, depression, attention deficit disorder, and bipolar disorder. Schizophrenia is less common, but very serious. Eating disorders are another category. Personality disorders are yet another type.

Depression

Let's start with depression. Depression is a symptom and it is an illness. I can detect depression from the energy level of my patient, the facial expressions, and appearance. A simple nine-question test called the PHQ-9 (Patient Health Questionnaire-9) is a validated screener for depression. It's available free online at www.phqscreeners.com and I have all my patients complete this form at their annual physical. I also have anyone presenting with mental health issues, and anyone on antidepressant medication, complete it. Under 5 points is normal, 6–10 is often mild depression. 11–15 moderate, and 16 and over may be a severe depression. Depression can be a mood, a feeling, but it can also manifest with low physical energy, eating too much or too little, sleep changes, or lack of interest in usual activities or grooming.

The first thing here is to make the diagnosis. I can't help a patient if I don't recognize they are suffering from depression. This is why continuity with your primary care doctor, your family doctor is important. When I see a patient for five, ten, fifteen years and they come in looking and acting differently, it is obvious to me. Less so with someone I don't know as well, although with the PHQ-9 test and listening to the patient, the diagnosis can be made.

Everyone is aware of anti-depressant medication, but my first go-to is psychology. This can be journaling, or writing about feelings. This can be a referral to a great therapist that I work with. Usually individual therapy is the best route for depression, at least initially. Depression is an opportunity to learn about yourself and to improve your life; it just doesn't feel like that at the time you are depressed. Medication plus therapy works better than either alone for moderate to severe depression. Certainly medication alone is the least expensive way to help someone who is depressed. But therapy can be really important for feeling better and for growing as a person and living better in the future.

First-line medication options include escitalopram (Lexapro) an SSRI (serotonin reuptake inhibitor) medication, or venlafaxine (Effexor), an SNRI (serotonin/norepinephrine medication). When anxiety is also present, I go with the SSRI, either escitalopram or sertraline (Zoloft). Both work well on depression and anxiety. I start with low dosages on these medications. Escitalopram comes with a lowest dose of 5 mg. I start with that dosage. I will even have some smaller patients (under 130 lbs) start with ½ of the dose (by cutting the small pill in half) and then increase after a week or two to 5 mg.

Some people respond well to 5 mg, but when I see people back at about three weeks (video or in person), some need to be increased to 10 mg. I believe the trend is to use lower doses of these medications than ten years ago, and I have led that move in my own practice for years. I was taught in medical school—start low, go slow. It is a safe, effective approach for these kinds of conditions. (Note that for an infection, start high and reduce if appropriate; different situation, of course.)

People may respond in less than a week or it may take dosage raises or up to three weeks to see a significant response. Be patient, work with your doctor on this.

Depression is a common medical condition. There is no shame in having depression, and it is diagnosable and treatable. Treatment may consist of purely lifestyle changes or therapy. Commonly, medication plus therapy is used and gets the best results. Psychiatry can be involved for complex cases or when a family doctor has used the common tools and seeks more advanced options. (see end of chapter for a self-screening form)

Psychiatry's Role

Psychiatrists are primarily psychopharmacologists and complex condition diagnosticians. They focus on the medications and the combinations of medications. So I involve a psychiatrist when a patient is not responding to my first-line medication, or perhaps my second choice, or where someone may be suicidal, or when they might have a more complicated diagnosis like bipolar disorder. Another reasonable reason for referral is dual diagnosis or uncertain diagnosis.

An experienced, well-trained family doctor can initiate and manage many cases of depression often with the help of a therapist.

Anxiety

How about anxiety? This problem is common, even growing in the younger population, post-Covid. Like depression, we want to consider alternatives to pills. Assessment includes a history of symptoms (interestingly, most are physical—fast heart beat, palpitations, sweating, shaking, etc.). A GAD-7 screening questionnaire can be somewhat helpful, especially in assessing progress or lack thereof with treatment recommendations.

Exercise is a great treatment to reduce anxiety (and it also helps depression). Cardio is the key, and 30 minutes minimum a day is usually a recommended amount. Meditation can also be helpful. Start with five minutes and build up to 15 minutes a day, slowly, if you can. The type of meditation doesn't matter. You can learn meditation from YouTube videos and lots of great websites.

Breathing exercises can also help, especially acutely. "Square" breathing is one example. Four seconds you breathe in, four seconds you hold, four seconds out, and four seconds wait. Repeat. The timing is like a square, equal sides. You can do three seconds if four seems too long.

4–7–8 breathing is another. Breathe slowly for four seconds. Hold for seven seconds (less if you are more comfortable), then breathe out through your nose (or mouth) very slowly for eight seconds. All of these breathing techniques encourage you to ultimately breathe more slowly. This activates the vagus nerve and relaxes us. Most of us breathe 12–14 times a minute. So either of these breathing techniques, done for a minute or two, takes us down closer to 3–5 breaths per minute. There are even devices to help you learn to breathe more slowly. If you feel lightheaded, short of breath, etc. **do not** follow these patterns and just regulate your breath slightly more slowly than usual.

Benzos vs. SSRIs

Beyond behavioral techniques, we have moved more toward preventive medication than as-needed medications. The as-needed fall into the benzo category like Lorazepam or Klonopin and would be used when anxiety strikes intensely. They take a while to work if swallowed, work much faster if allowed to dissolve under the tongue. But again the anxiety or panic attack has already happened, so we are treating it during or after the fact. Most docs prefer to prescribe a medication like the SSRIs mentioned above—escitalopram or sertraline—as a medication that is taken daily can, within a few weeks, dramatically reduce anxiety and keep it under control. Dosages tend to be lower than moderate to severe depression, and I start low on these and only go up if needed. Combining the behavioral approaches above with the medications is often the best approach. Follow-up in the office or video is important to ensure relief and to fine-tune the approach, check in about stressors in the patient's life, and monitor dosages.

Attention Deficit Disorder

While this is perceived as mostly a condition of children, ADD and ADHD can also affect adults. This includes many of the individuals who had ADHD as a child. It's more common in men than women. Some people are able to "grow out of it". Some develop behavioral workarounds in terms of when they work, distractions, white noise, bursts of activity, etc.

Some come to the office afraid of losing their job or of failing out of a graduate program after returning to school after many years. There is an excellent self-assessment tool called the Adult ADHD Self-Report Scale (ASRS-v1.1) that I use with patients to help diagnose the condition. This validated questionnaire is available online and can help identify symptoms of adult ADHD. Some already come in diagnosed by a prior neuropsychologist or psychiatrist, and with these, the diagnosis is not the issue. The Adult ADHD Self-Report (ASRS) is available: www.hcp.med.harvard.edu/ncs/asrs.php

I do a urine toxicology test in the office. Mixing these medications with illicit drugs like cocaine or PCP can be very dangerous, so I emphasize sobriety from these agents. THC (marijuana, cannabis) is not a concern, nor is social alcohol use. The medications I will prescribe for ADHD are stimulants. The interesting part is that if someone without ADHD takes these medications, they often feel uncomfortable, wired, hyper, and don't want to take them. Someone with ADHD tends to feel focused, clear, organized. Our nervous systems are built differently. People with ADHD seem to need this stimulation to a part of the brain that allows them to regulate their focus and attention.

My go-to medication is Adderall (mixed amphetamine salts) although there are alternatives that are also good (Ritalin, Concerta, Dextroamphetamine, etc.). I start with 5 or 10 mg, and the patient usually uses them first thing in the morning on the way to work, and may need an early afternoon dose to get through the latter part of the workday. Some patients skip on the weekends entirely, which is great, and allows them to relax and be social without the focus. Others might take it for errands on one weekend day and skip the other weekend doses. I do allow patients to skip during the week as well. It's not like an antidepressant where you have to take it daily exactly as prescribed. I had one patient who took it to do paperwork, but skipped it for sales calls which were more open-ended, enjoyable for her, and social. There are extended-release versions of this medication, once a patient is stable and comfortable with use.

Some patients need these medications to work and to function for years. Others develop the skills to compensate for their tendency to mentally wander or find creative fields where it's less of an issue. I monitor heart rate and blood pressure at every visit. Sometimes heart rates go up; rarely is blood pressure affected. I randomly monitor urine for toxicology throughout the year and do find the occasional positive cocaine test, which leads me to stop prescribing the medication until the urine is clear and the usually contrite individual commits to a sober lifestyle and frequent testing until I am convinced it's no longer a problem.

Vyvanse is another option, longer lasting, smoother release of medication. Some patients thrive on it, others not so much. Adderall XR (extended release) is another option that may be less expensive. Taken once a day, there is again, no need to take a second dose in the afternoon, and the effect is smoother throughout the day.

Doctor's Note: *Mental health is health. Depression and anxiety are medical conditions, not character flaws. Treatment works—whether through therapy, medication, or both. Don't suffer in silence; reach out and get the help you need… and deserve.*

Here is a **PHQ-9 with scoring**. If you score high, bring this to your physician's attention soon. If you have any suicidal thoughts or plans, call your doctor or a suicide hotline immediately.

This is from Washington State's public website.

	Over the last 2 weeks, how often have you been bothered by the following problems?	Not at all	Several Days	More than half the days	Nearly every day
1	Little interest or pleasure in doing things	0	1	2	3
2	Feeling down, depressed, or hopeless	0	1	2	3
3	Trouble falling asleep or sleeping too much	0	1	2	3
4	Feeling tired or having little energy	0	1	2	3
5	Poor appetite or overeating	0	1	2	3
6	Feeling bad about yourself- or that you are a failure or have let yourself or family down	0	1	2	3
7	Trouble concentrating on things, such as reading the newspaper or watching television	0	1	2	3
8	Moving or speaking so slowly that other people could have noticed. Or the opposite-being so fidgety or restless that you have been moving around a lot more than usual	0	1	2	3
9	Thoughts that you would be better off dead, or of hurting yourself in some way	0	1	2	3
	TOTAL SCORE (add the marked numbers):				

How to score the PHQ-9

1. Assign scores: For each of the nine questions, assign the corresponding number:
   - Not at all = 0
   - Several days = 1
   - More than half the days = 2
   - Nearly every day = 3

2. Sum the scores: Add up the points from all nine questions to get a total score, which can range from 0 to 27.

3. Interpret the score: Use the total score to determine the severity of depression and the recommended next steps:
   - 0–4: Minimal depression. No action needed, rescreen annually.
   - 5–9: Mild depression. Watchful waiting, consider repeating the PHQ-9 at a follow-up appointment.
   - 10–14: Moderate depression. Develop a treatment plan that may include counseling, follow-up, or pharmacotherapy.
   - 15–19: Moderately severe depression. Initiate active treatment with pharmacotherapy and/or psychotherapy.
   - 20+: Severe depression. Start immediate pharmacotherapy and consider an expedited referral to a mental health specialist.

CHAPTER 24

DIABETES MELLITUS

The vast majority of diabetes diagnosed in adults is Type II. This is the adult-onset type, related to metabolism, diet, genetics, and weight. Type I diabetes more commonly occurs in children and is associated with a lack of insulin, hence insulin injections are usually required. Type II is related to reduced insulin sensitivity at the tissue level and other factors. There can be a mixed Type I-II diabetes as well.

Diabetes mellitus means 'sweet urine,' referring to the glucose that spills into urine. The condition is caused by decreased sensitivity to insulin in the tissues (type II) or decreased insulin production (Type I). Most physicals and general checkups that include a blood test include a chemistry panel. Glucose is one of the values measured. Diabetes is diagnosed from either an elevated fasting glucose (above 125), an elevated random glucose (above 200), or most commonly and more accurately, an elevated HbA1c test (hemoglobin A1c). This test is able to measure the average glucose level over the prior three months. It measures the glucose attached to red cells, which live on average, about three months. Normal values are below 5.7.

Prediabetes is defined by an A1c between 5.7 and 6.4. Diabetes is determined by an A1c 6.5 or above. Obviously, the higher the value (7, 8, 9), the more serious or more poorly controlled the condition is. For prediabetes, which is statistically very common in an adult population (and increasingly in children and adolescents), the initial treatment is usually dietary changes combined with more aerobic exercise. Weight loss may also be valuable.

The A1c in prediabetes might be repeated in three to six months. If improving or normalized, the approach is continued. A dietician may be valuable to teach and guide a patient to the right types and quantities of food. Lowering carbohydrate intake (bread, cake, rice, potatoes) is often a key part of the diet, but not the only component. Having protein with each meal or snack (including nuts, tofu, eggs, cottage cheese, and fish or meat) seems to also moderate glucose spikes.

The next step in treatment could be medication. Metformin is the first line for most patients with diabetes or worsening prediabetes. This inexpensive, generic medication lowers glucose and may help some people to lose weight. Some studies have suggested anti-aging properties independent of diabetes and this is a potential added benefit. I advise ramping up the dose slowly as this medication can cause gastrointestinal upset or diarrhea in many individuals, especially as they begin treatment.

Another interesting option is continuous glucose monitoring (CGM), which is gradually replacing fingerstick glucose testing. CGM involves a patch placed on the skin with a tiny sensor that passes through the skin and measures capillary glucose levels, continuously. The patient typically reads the result on a phone app or separate device. This allows feedback as to which foods spike the glucose and which do not. This helps patients to maintain a healthy glucose level in their bloodstream. The device is covered by many insurance plans, but sometimes restricted to more severe cases. Costs are coming down for self-pay usage.

As a family doctor, I take care of pre-diabetes, mild diabetes, and typically involve an endocrinologist for more severe cases.

Doctor's Note: *Diabetes is a common medical condition. Diagnosing it early is important, ideally at a pre-diabetic stage. The A1c test is the most valuable blood test in this regard. There are effective lifestyle changes and medications to control or significantly improve the condition, particularly when caught early.*

CHAPTER 25

THYROID DISEASE

Many patients come in wondering if their thyroid function is abnormal. These are typically individuals who are overweight, sometimes underweight, or have trouble losing weight they wish to lose. Interestingly, a surprisingly small percentage of these individuals end up with a thyroid diagnosis. The thyroid gland regulates body metabolism. There is a complex interaction between the pituitary gland and the thyroid gland to regulate the proper release of hormones into the system.

We start by examining the thyroid gland in the neck for enlargement, nodules or masses. Blood tests might include a TSH (Thyroid stimulating hormone), a free T3, free T4 (free indicates not bound to blood proteins), and sometimes other tests as well. We may test for antibodies to the thyroid which can cause conditions including Hashimoto's Disease (an autoimmune type of thyroid inflammation).

If the labs are normal, the patient does not have clinically evident thyroid disease. If the doctor feels a nodule or mass, the next step might be an ultrasound of the thyroid. Typically small cysts can be determined to be benign and followed with another ultrasound in a year. Larger cysts might require aspiration by a specialist or radiologist. Masses might require other types of imaging. Thyroid cancer is actually somewhat common and usually very effectively treated and often cured.

A goiter is an enlarged thyroid. Symptoms can include a hoarse voice or difficulty swallowing. Typically benign, it can also be cosmetically noticeable. Treatment depends on the cause and the size and typically involves medications or rarely surgery. Thyroid levels are tested and often low doses of thyroid hormone may help the goiter to recede in size or return to normal. Sometimes a goiter may precede a thyroid condition such as hypothyroidism (low thyroid function) or be related to inflammation from an inflammatory condition.

On the other hand, there is also hyperthyroidism. This condition is caused by an overactive thyroid gland, and classically is associated with weight loss, anxiety, and even heart rhythm abnormalities. For example, a man with new onset atrial fibrillation should be tested for an overactive thyroid with lab tests. Graves' disease is one type. This condition may be associated with prominent eyeballs (proptosis is the medical description). It is usually autoimmune.

Doctor's Note: *The thyroid gland is important in metabolism. Testing the gland's function with blood tests is simple. If there is a growth, ultrasound or other imaging is done to determine if a benign cyst or something else. Both underactive and overactive thyroid conditions are diagnosable and treatable. Thyroid cancer, if found, is often effectively treated.*

CHAPTER 26

ASTHMA AND COPD

Asthma is a common respiratory condition where there is inflammation of the airways and spasm of the bronchial tubes. It can present in childhood and disappear, or present in adulthood, sometimes triggered by bronchitis, and persist or recur. Sometimes the condition and the need for treatment is lifelong. A related condition is COPD (chronic obstructive pulmonary disease) which usually occurs as we age and can be related to smoking and occupational exposures. This condition can be quite severe, at times, and needs appropriate treatment. Difficult breathing, shortness of breath, and wheezing are some of the symptoms with both asthma and COPD.

The typical first line therapy for asthma is an albuterol inhaler. This is also known as a "rescue inhaler" because it works quickly and its effects may last four to six hours. Brand names include ProAir, Ventolin, and others. A person whose asthma is triggered by exercise which is called EIA (Exercise-induced asthma) may find that using the inhaler fifteen to thirty minutes before exercise is very effective in increasing lung capacity and making breathing easier. Olympic athletes need special permission, therefore, to use this medication if they have an actual diagnosis of asthma.

But, asthma is also and perhaps primarily, an inflammatory condition of the airways. Thus, steroid-based inhalers that reduce inflammation, or sometimes oral medications (like prednisone) can also be used to effectively treat asthma and prevent or reduce frequency of attacks. Some brand names include Advair, Qvar, Pulmicort, Asmanex. They contain fluticasone and related corticosteroid medications. It is very important that these medications actually reach the lungs. Watching videos, talking to the pharmacist, practicing, and sometimes a spacer device help ensure this occurs. The spacer is a hollow plastic tube with openings at each end. The inhaler is fitted into one opening and sprayed into the chamber. One's mouth goes over the other opening and when breathing it, it is easier to get all the medication into your lungs.

COPD treatment always involves smoking cessation. Long-acting bronchodilators are often prescribed. Key options include tiotropium (Spiriva), umeclidinium (Incruse), salmeterol (Serevent), and indacaterol (Arcapta). For more severe cases and for difficult-to-control or complex COPD, I involve a pulmonary specialist in the patient's care. Mild cases and exacerbations, I am usually able to provide treatment for, or if after hours, urgent care centers do a good job as well.

Doctor's Note: *Asthma is common. Medications are available to treat and even prevent exacerbations. Technique is important with inhalers; spacer devices may help. COPD, often related to smoking, requires its own management plan and specialist involvement in more advanced cases.*

CHAPTER 27
OSTEOPOROSIS

Osteoporosis, or thinning and weakening of the bones, occurs as we age. The key is to start off with as much bone as possible and then to manage the decline well. This can be said of most of aging, as well. Softer bones are more likely to break and fractures in the spine can affect our posture and height, as well as be painful. Fractures in our hips can be even more devastating, often requiring surgery, and prolonged rehabilitation.

We reach our maximal bone density by about age 30. 90% of that occurs by age 20. So it is important to be active as a child, climbing, running, throwing, etc. Kids move naturally, we just need to give them the opportunity at home and at school. Continue weight bearing exercises in your 20's and ideally throughout your life to maximize bone as you build and slow the decline that typically starts at age 40 or 50. These include walking, hiking, running, weight lifting and body weight exercises—pushups, etc. Swimming is fantastic but as we are buoyant in the water, there may be less bone building than other land sports.

Above 60, we may start checking a patient for bone density with a DEXA scan. This is a low intensity x-ray scan. By low intensity, I mean that the technician can stay in the room while you are being tested and very little radiation is utilized. The scan often focuses on the lumbar spine, hip, and a particular area of the hip in more detail. The results are reviewed by a radiologist and a report is issued to the ordering physician. Family doctors can order this test.

Rheumatologists do as well and sometimes act as specialists for abnormal findings. For mild changes, like osteopenia, typically diet is discussed such as getting sufficient calcium (1000–1200 mg a day). This can be dietary or supplements or both. Exercise as discussed above is also advised. Finally, vitamin D3 supplements are a co-factor which can help strengthen bone along with the calcium.

For more severe changes, the category of osteoporosis, there are both oral medications such as Fosamax and injectable or intravenous infusions such as Prolia or Reclast (zoledronic acid). The advantage of infusions is less frequent administration and perhaps fewer GI effects than oral medications. Discuss with your doctor what is best for you and your case. This is always done along with diet and supplements, where appropriate.

There are some risks to these medications, including dental problems, so the decision to go on medications should be carefully considered. With good oral hygiene, the dental risk is quite low. Sometimes a second opinion is helpful in sorting this out.

Repeat scans are often done every two years, where appropriate. Note that some illnesses such as malabsorption or celiac disease, family history of severe osteoporosis, may necessitate earlier screening with DEXA scans.

Doctor's Note: *Strong bones are important, especially as we age. Building up bone density with weight bearing exercise, when younger, helps a lot. Dietary intake of calcium and vitamin D3 via sunshine and supplement is also of benefit. Medications are typically used when the condition of the bones is at risk for fracture, a condition called osteoporosis.*

CHAPTER 28

HORMONES AND MENOPAUSE

My female patients all have gynecologists; I haven't performed gynecological exams or pap smears for several decades. But, hormone replacement therapy does come up with them, as it does with male patients.

Menopause typically occurs between ages 48 and 54, when estrogen and progesterone production diminishes and menstrual cycles cease. Peri-menopause begins about five years earlier. A woman is defined as having gone through menopause when she has not had a period for a year.

During my career, I have seen trends occur where everyone was on hormone replacement at menopause to almost no one, to quite a significant number today. Some of this was based upon concern, stemming from studies suggesting that the benefits of estrogen were outweighed by risks. The benefits include reducing or eliminating hot flashes, feeling better overall, improved bone density, reduced risk of cardiovascular disease, and improved vaginal health and sexual function. Progesterone, the other main female hormone, may help with sleep and other functions.

Theoretical risks of hormone replacement include endometrial cancer, which can be monitored for fairly easily. Office testing such as transvaginal ultrasound or a simple transvaginal endometrial biopsy procedure can determine if any problems exist. Also,

an increased risk of breast cancer **was** believed to be a consideration, although more recent studies suggest this is not a significant risk. Obviously, mammograms and screenings are routinely advised in women of this age group. Combined therapy with progesterone reduces the risk of endometrial cancer, but may cause women to bleed intermittently. Women without a uterus are typically treated with estrogen alone.

Some women are also prescribed small amounts of testosterone as part of a hormone replacement program. Their levels are tested and this may be helpful if reduced libido is a significant factor for them.

These medications are available as pills, creams, and patches. Transdermal patches (through the skin) offer absorption benefits, particularly for estrogen and testosterone. Typically progesterone is given orally.

Doctor's Note: *I defer to my gynecology colleagues on the specifics, but currently, many patients benefit from hormone replacement in a variety of ways, with risks that are lower than once believed.*

SECTION 6

Medications and Treatments

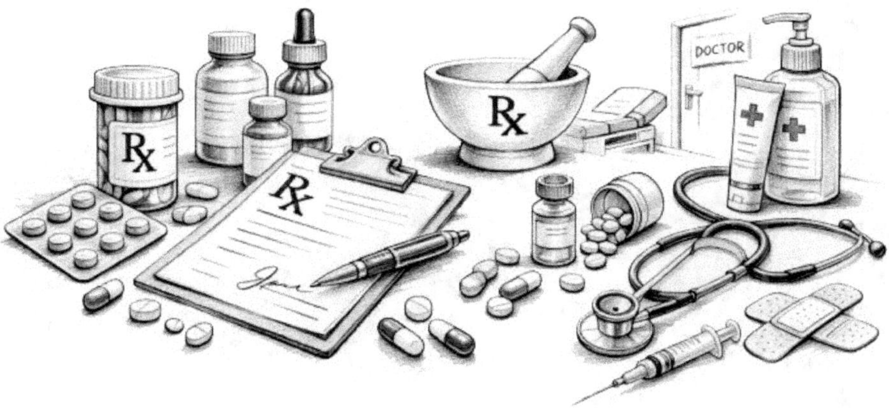

CHAPTER 29

Common Over-the-Counter Medications

These are medications you can purchase without a prescription, directly from a pharmacy or some mail order services (Amazon, others).

Voltaren Gel

For musculoskeletal and sports injuries, Diclofenac gel (Voltaren gel) is a very helpful and important item to have in the home. I have known about this topical medication for over 30 years, although it came to the US as a prescription medication only in 2007. In 2020, it went over the counter. Voltaren is widely known around the world as an effective anti-inflammatory medication (with the usual caveats about oral consumption including risks of GI side effects, gastritis, ulcers, etc.). The topical has big advantages because it is minimally absorbed in the bloodstream and therefore the risks are dramatically lower.

Some injuries are very superficial. Some are deeper. Diclofenac gel, or any topical, is going to be more effective for the superficial ones. To name a few, biceps tendonitis—helpful, labral tear—much less so. Wrist tendinitis—helpful. Tennis elbow—helpful. Deep gluteal strain—less so. Use common sense. Follow instructions for use. Typically I have patients squeeze some onto the last segment of their index finger and rub it in well three to four times a day. It can be a little greasy, so some soak-in time or a shirt you don't care much about is a wise choice.

Acetaminophen (Tylenol)

Acetaminophen (Tylenol) is a remarkable medication and very effective for fever, many types of pain, and fever with malaise (feeling lousy). It is my personal go-to for viral infections. Follow dosage instructions for your age and weight. About 15 mg/kg of weight is reasonable. I take 1000 mg and get eight great hours of relief when I am ill. Try to avoid using it more than three times a day and use it for brief periods of time.

Guidelines suggest risk is significant for liver issues above 4000 mg a day, with risks at 3000 mg for extended periods and even 2000 mg in the elderly and smaller people. My personal dosage of 1000 mg three times a day (exactly eight hours apart) is 3000 mg a day. If you use 650 mg three or four times a day, you are well below 3000 mg in a day. Very effective medication with no known GI risks. Interesting studies have suggested that acetaminophen may reduce 'social pain' or emotional distress—a form of psychological discomfort. This may explain why it's particularly effective for the overall malaise that comes with illness. Physical and psychological distress are closely related. A preliminary study suggested that it may even reduce existential anxiety!

NSAIDs

Ibuprofen, naproxen (Advil, Aleve) are NSAIDs. Non-steroidal anti-inflammatory medications (NSAIDs). This is to contrast them with steroidal anti-inflammatory meds which include prednisone, Medrol, cortisone, etc. NSAIDs are great for pain, headaches, menstrual cramps, and fever. They reduce inflammation, although the most anti-inflammatory benefit comes with prolonged usage at higher dosing. You get mostly pain and fever relief at lower dosages. The bottles suggest that one 200 mg ibuprofen every four to six hours can help. Or one naproxen every eight to twelve hours.

But as a physician, I always advise higher dosages, ideally for shorter intervals. So 400–800 mg ibuprofen depending on size (that 15 milligrams per kilogram rule is reasonable here, too.) Typically three times a day with food. Or two naproxen every twelve hours, again with food Taking these medications with food significantly reduces the risk of GI irritation, but does not eliminate it. There are many other anti-inflammatory medications that are prescription only and have the advantage of being only once a day or at most twice, making the usage simpler for people.

The principal risk of NSAIDs is kidney damage. This is far more likely with prolonged use, especially at higher doses. So use these cautiously beyond a few weeks, although with medical supervision, many patients take them for longer. Blood tests, for example, for renal function can be checked by your doctor if you need to take them for a long period of time (e.g. more than three months).

Heartburn and GERD Medications

Heartburn, GERD, and sour stomach meds include famotidine (Pepcid) and omeprazole (Prilosec). Famotidine is an H-2 medication, very safe, and reasonably effective for occasional use for acid-related symptoms. It reduces acid production in the stomach lining. Similarly, omeprazole is effective: it's a different category, a PPI (proton pump inhibitor) medication, and blocks acid production and symptoms from the same. The key here is when to realize that you're not getting adequate relief from the OTC options and seeing a physician for further assessment. If you find yourself taking these daily or an increasing amount per week, then consult with your family doctor. Sometimes, stronger medications are appropriate. Sometimes further testing or a gastroenterology (GI) consultation is indicated. PPI medications were designed for shorter term use although many patients do need to take them for longer periods. Discuss this with your doctor.

I should also mention calcium carbonate tablets (TUMS) which are rapidly effective for heartburn and sour stomach. Great to have some with you if you're prone to this after rich meals or some alcohol. These work very quickly. This or equivalent is even used in the emergency room to help differentiate chest pain from acid versus chest pain from the heart. Again, don't diagnose yourself, if you are concerned about heart attack symptoms or angina, get checked out. But if you are a worrier, and get some chest pain that is likely acid related, warm water or taking TUMS should clarify the issue quickly. As with the above medications, if you are using this daily or with increased frequency, see your family doctor for assessment and medication options.

Allergy Meds

The allergy medications are over the counter (used to be prescription). Loratadine (Claritin) is my favorite, but Zyrtec (cetirizine) and Allegra (fexofenadine) are also popular and effective. These are amazing in comparison to older allergy options because they are mostly non-sedating. The Benadryl (diphenhydramine) and Chlortrimeton (chlorpheniramine) days led to a lot of sleepiness and inability to function. Most of the modern ones are once a day and help with seasonal allergies and work fairly quickly for mild allergic reactions to bee stings, plant irritation, food allergies, and the like. However, if you are having issues with breathing (anaphylaxis), an Epipen (epinephrine injectable) and an emergency room visit are essential.

Allergy diagnosis and treatment are advancing, and the use of sublingual immunotherapy (SLIT) in some cases is intriguing. Administered at home, although mixed up by an allergist or pharmacist, this treatment avoids allergy shots which involve visits to the doctor's office with time associated.

Skin Creams

Hydrocortisone over-the-counter cream is great for itching and for many rashes coming from dry skin or allergies. Rashes from fungus respond well to OTC Lotrimin (clotrimazole). Sometimes you are not sure, and should see your family doctor to get a clear direction or prescription medication. Dermatologists play a role if you already have one or if your primary care doctor is unsure of a diagnosis or treatment.

Lidocaine (Xylocaine), a local anesthetic, comes in patches and creams designed to relieve pain. Sometimes combined with other agents such as in sunburn medication, and other times in OTC creams or patches or higher-strength Rx patches. Symptomatic relief is the goal here; lidocaine doesn't fix something, but it does help you to feel better and perhaps ignore the area for a while, which can have brain benefits (see prior pain section) and therefore help with healing. The prescription version lidocaine film patch is used for 12 hours a day and you can choose which twelve hour window to use it. It is kept off the other twelve hours of the day to avoid toxicity reactions. My patients with night pain put it on at 9 or 10 p.m.; my patients with day pain put it on when they awaken. Twelve hours later, remove the patch.

Nasal Issues

For nasal congestion, oxymetazoline (Afrin) nasal spray is effective in opening your nasal passages for twelve hours. I strongly advise not to use it for more than 3–4 days as the rebound effect can lead people to more stuffiness. This occurs after using it too long, and this can lead to a form of habituation, where people use the spray to relieve the stuffiness they get from having stopped using it. The solution is to add fluticasone (Flonase) to the Afrin during the 3–4 days and then continue the safe Flonase spray once or twice a day. Flonase does not produce as dramatic a response as Afrin, but its anti-inflammatory properties reduce stuffiness longer term, work on allergies and cold-related symptoms and are generally safe.

Nasal Irrigation

An over-the-counter treatment I love is nasal irrigation. The big brand here is NeilMed. Is this a Neti Pot I am referring to? Well, that is one way to administer saline to the nose and sinuses. But a more modern and I believe more effective and easier-to-use method is the squeeze bottles that NeilMed (and other companies) make. This is not nasal mist. This is flushing saline through your nose up into your sinuses and out the other side. The bottle is about eight ounces, so it takes 2–3 times each side to rinse.

I do it myself for allergies, every single day, and I find a lot of twisting, turning side-to-side and head-down posture over the sink ensures that every drop of saline comes out during the process and not two hours later in the gym! Very effective, seems to reduce allergy symptoms, help with colds, even knock off some early sinus infections before they can take hold. Use it daily as prevention, and to flush dust, pollen, pollution, and even viruses—out of your nasal passageways before they do harm. Also use it once or twice a day, along with steamy showers or steam inhalation, during acute episodes of upper respiratory infection and sinusitis.

Doctor's Note: *Over-the-counter doesn't mean risk-free. Use these medications wisely—follow dosing instructions, know what you're taking, and recognize when it's time to see your doctor. Many OTC options are highly effective when used correctly.*

CHAPTER 30

COMMON PRESCRIPTION MEDICATIONS

Just like the over-the-counter section has way too many options to discuss all of them, prescription medications are their own course in medical school. This is not a pharmacology textbook, so let's just hit some highlights.

Recent data suggest these are the twenty most commonly prescribed medications in the US; let's go over each one briefly, and I'll extend my comments where I believe it would be helpful to do so.

1. Levothyroxine (for thyroid conditions)
2. Atorvastatin (for high cholesterol)
3. Metformin (for type 2 diabetes)
4. Lisinopril (for high blood pressure and heart conditions)
5. Amlodipine (for high blood pressure and heart conditions)
6. Amoxicillin (antibiotic)
7. Vitamin D supplements (for deficiency)
8. Amphetamine/dextroamphetamine (for ADHD)
9. Omeprazole (for acid reflux and ulcers)
10. Gabapentin (for nerve pain and epilepsy)
11. Sertraline (antidepressant)
12. Hydrochlorothiazide (diuretic for high blood pressure)
13. Metoprolol (for high blood pressure and heart conditions)

14. Escitalopram (antidepressant)
15. Albuterol (for asthma and COPD)
16. Losartan (for high blood pressure)
17. Bupropion (antidepressant)
18. Furosemide (diuretic)
19. Pantoprazole (for acid reflux and ulcers)
20. Trazodone (antidepressant and sleep aid)

1. Levothyroxine (for thyroid conditions). For people diagnosed with low thyroid function through laboratory testing, this is the go-to medication to replace what we naturally produce with a synthetic version. People on this medication are monitored more frequently initially and then once a year is usually enough for stable patients. It is often a lifetime medication, but well tolerated in most people. Brand name: Synthroid

2. Atorvastatin (for high cholesterol)—The statin category of medications has contributed to a reduced rate of heart attacks and strokes in the US over the last forty years. Obviously, lifestyle factors and approaches are also important in high cholesterol and vascular disease management as well. I have discussed cardiac screening tests earlier. If you have a need for this medication, the vast majority of patients find it easy to tolerate. A small number of people are switched to other statins (of which there are 7–8 approved in the US) or an alternative non-statin medication. There are now some injectable options, given weekly, monthly, or less often for some people with severe cases or more significant vascular disease that represent a new frontier for treatment. Brand Name: Lipitor

3. Metformin (for type 2 diabetes). Despite all the diabetes medications available, metformin remains the

guideline-approved choice for the first medication to use in Type 2 diabetes and some cases of prediabetes as well. Metformin may cause mild GI side effects which usually improve with time. Some people lose some weight on the medication, which is usually desirable. Monitoring the A1c blood test is crucial to dosing the medication effectively. Exercise and good dietary intake are also important here. Brand Name: Glucophage

4. Lisinopril (for high blood pressure and heart conditions) The most commonly prescribed ACE inhibitor (angiotensin converting enzyme) is an effective, and usually well-tolerated blood pressure medication effective as a first-line choice in most people. This may not be as effective in African American patients; other meds may work better. The major side effect of this medication is a dry cough, in about 5 percent of people. If this occurs, and it can be subtle and confusing, then we switch to a different, related category of blood pressure meds (ARB meds, see #16 below) and the cough resolves. Brand Names: Zestril, Prinivil

5. Amlodipine (for high blood pressure and heart conditions) A calcium blocker medication that affects calcium in the blood vessel, not the blood circulation. So your calcium level is not affected, but your blood pressure is. Usually an effective medication, often used in conjunction with another BP medication, as a second line medication. Many patients with blood pressure require two meds; some need three for BP control. A side effect of leg swelling can be annoying and sometimes leads to reducing the dosage or changing the medication entirely. Brand Name: Norvasc

6. Amoxicillin (antibiotic) Oldie but a goodie. I use antibiotics sparingly. Most upper respiratory infections are viral. Also,

there are urinary infections and sinus infections resistant to amoxicillin, so I tend to use Augmentin (amoxicillin plus clavulanic acid) more often when I do prescribe. Doxycycline and Bactrim (trimethoprim-sulfamethoxazole) are two other generic but effective antibiotics that I prescribe when needed.

7. Vitamin D supplements Generally OTC is fine here. The higher-dose supplements that are taken once a week are prescription. I believe it's more physiologic to take a lower dose daily. For example, instead of 50,000 units once a week for severe deficiency, take 5000 units daily and double up on Tuesday and Sunday.

8. Amphetamine/dextroamphetamine (for ADHD) aka Adderall is an effective medication for people with attention/focus disorders. Used more commonly in adults, it was once just a kids' medication. Proper selection of patients, starting with low dosages, and consideration for behavioral approaches to managing ADD/ADHD are all appropriate.

9. Omeprazole (for acid reflux and ulcers) Discussed previously in its OTC incarnation. It comes in higher dosages by prescription (as do a number of other OTC meds) Brand Name: Prilosec

10. Gabapentin (for nerve pain and epilepsy) Initially developed for seizures, this medication has remarkable versatility with benefits for nerve pain, mood disorders, sleep, and other nervous system conditions. Dosing is tricky, and many patients do well with low doses for sleep, although for chronic nerve pain, much higher dosages, with gradual up-titration of dose, are needed and tolerated. If started on too much, too soon, side effects can limit its use. Brand Name: Neurontin

11. Sertraline (antidepressant) Effective SSRI (serotonin reuptake inhibitor) medication for depression and anxiety. Perhaps used more for anxiety than any other antidepressant, and avoids the addictive properties of benzodiazepines in that regard. Start low and build up to an effective dosage as tolerated. Some people do great on very low doses, especially for anxiety. Side effects vary, more common in higher dosing, and can include reduced libido. Brand Name: Zoloft

12. Hydrochlorothiazide (diuretic for high blood pressure) A water pill, or diuretic,—works by helping us excrete excess fluid from our system. Hence, avoid taking before bedtime. Often used along with ACE or ARB medications as a BP team approach. Rarely used alone anymore. Monitor sodium, potassium, and other electrolytes on this medication. Eating enough potassium-containing foods (e.g. bananas) may be enough for most patients; some may need potassium supplement after measuring lab tests.

13. Metoprolol (for high blood pressure and heart conditions) Most commonly prescribed beta-blocker medication that controls blood pressure, regulates heart rate (slows it somewhat). Usually well tolerated, by starting low and building up, fatigue and other effects are diminished. Often used with other BP medications. May be used after a heart attack to reduce risk of another. May have a slightly calming effect as do other beta blockers, at least by making us less aware of, or having less of, a racing heart rate, sweaty palms, etc. Brand Name: Toprol

14. Escitalopram (antidepressant) Commonly prescribed SSRI medication with benefits for depression and anxiety. Weight gain is not uncommon and needs to be managed

effectively, or people may wish to stop the medication, even if their mood improves. Effective in low doses for anxiety and depression, with dosing often lower for anxiety. The smallest pill is 5 mg (highest 20 mg) and I sometimes start people on ½ of the 5 mg, i.e. 2.5 mg. Brand Name: Lexapro

15. Albuterol (for asthma and COPD) is the essential ingredient in most asthma inhalers and some for COPD (chronic obstructive pulmonary disease). The most common method of use is the aerosol inhaler, sometimes called a puffer, and timing and technique are important in getting the medication to the lungs, not the mouth and oropharynx. Brand Names: Proventil, Ventolin, ProAir

16. Losartan (for high blood pressure) The most commonly prescribed in the ARB category (angiotensin receptor blocker). Few side effects, well tolerated, effective, although like other BP meds, may need to be used in conjunction with other medications in some patients. Brand Name: Cozaar

17. Bupropion (antidepressant) A stimulating antidepressant. Many of the antidepressants calm patients. This one can get someone out of a listless rut. Gets a patient moving along in their life. It can reduce the drive to smoke and other habits. It may be used in some cases along with another antidepressant. Starting low and building up is essential. May make some people more anxious than they would like to feel. But lacks the libido suppression of some medications so that is a big benefit with some patients. Brand Name: Wellbutrin

18. Furosemide (diuretic) A tubular diuretic; again, avoid taking before bedtime. Used for heart failure to reduce fluid

volume in the body. Monitor electrolytes, especially potassium, but also sodium and magnesium. Can be used for blood pressure as well, in low dosages, along with other medications in almost all cases. Brand Name: Lasix

19. Pantoprazole (for acid reflux and ulcers) Effective PPI (proton pump inhibitor) medication that is not over the counter. Some concerns with long-term usage, although many people are on it for long periods as GERD can be difficult to cure with other measures, and this medication controls symptoms and may reduce risks of chronic acid reflux on the esophagus. Brand Name: Protonix

20. Trazodone (antidepressant and sleep aid) Older serotonin-elevating antidepressant that has found a newer use as a sleep aid. In far lower dosages than its use for depression, people often fall asleep and stay asleep better. Far less habit-forming risk than benzos and Z-drugs (mentioned previously). Not perfect for sleep, and some people find benefits wearing off after a while. Brand Name: Desyrel

Doctor's Note: *These twenty medications treat some of the most common conditions I see. Understanding what you're taking and why helps you be an active partner in your care. Never hesitate to ask questions about your prescriptions. Sometimes with lifestyle changes or weight loss, medications can be deprescribed. That is gratifying for all concerned.*

CHAPTER 31

Alternative Medicine

I don't like the term "Alternative medicine." Alternative to what, I would ask. The term "integrative medicine" better captures the essence of combining what Western medical doctors learn in school—medication, surgery, lab testing, etc. and the best of Eastern and Indigenous Medicine, including acupuncture, chiropractic, and body work. I'm open to these approaches, and there is often a nuanced conversation about safety and expectations.

I answer questions and I do want to know if my patients are participating in treatments that I did not prescribe. Many do. Acupuncture is a system of treatment utilizing meridians on the body and a model of energy and organ involvement different from Western medicine or modern scientific understanding. But it works for many people. And it doesn't work for some. I have found the most benefit for acupuncture for conditions involving pain such as tennis elbow and headaches, although people use it for all kinds of medical conditions. Unlike physical therapy, you don't get stronger. So that's a deficit.

Many acupuncture doctors, trained in Chinese medicine, like to combine needles and herbal therapy. Here there can be a conflict. If my patient is on prescription medicine, I caution the use of herbs because we usually don't know the exact ingredients, and interactions between herbs and prescription medicine are common. If herbal medicine was not active medicine, it wouldn't help, so it makes sense that one needs to be aware of interactions.

However, given the difficulty of understanding these interaction risks and questions about the purity and safety of herbs ordered from abroad, I advise avoiding these, in general.

Chiropractic

Chiropractic is something I have had a fair amount of experience with. I was briefly medical director of an MD-Chiropractic company with clinics many years ago. I have shared an office suite with two chiropractors for many years. Here is what I learned. Some patients do great with chiropractic, especially for low back pain. Some chiropractors have great manual skills for understanding and fixing minor injuries and misalignments. I do not believe in prolonged chiropractic care. I also don't believe in perpetual physical therapy. A treatment is supposed to help within a reasonable time period. If not, move on to something else. That has been my treatment philosophy for most conditions. Unlike medicine, where a blood pressure of a certain elevation, will lead to nearly the same prescription from just about any MD, there is a great variation in what chiropractors know and what they do to treat patients.

Have you heard the term "'straight' chiropractor" vs. "mixer"? No, this has nothing to do with one's social life. A straight chiropractor typically just does spinal adjustments and leaves the rest to nature or home exercise or other practitioners. A mixer may combine modalities like heat, ultrasound, laser therapy, rolling massage table, manual massage, exercise, etc. in the treatment plan. A mixer is closer to a physical therapist. So you really need to understand who the chiropractor is who you are thinking of seeing. You need to understand what they do as well.

Some chiropractors, unfortunately, use x-rays to frighten patients into longer treatment schedules, even pre-paid programs. I do not find this medically logical or effective or ethically sound. Many of the findings they discuss with patients are seen equally in asymptomatic patients. Also, a treatment process should be guided by its effectiveness and changed when not effective. No one should commit to an expensive long process without knowing how they respond. Finally, some of these chiropractors have a model of incorporating expensive machinery based treatment like spinal traction into the package. This represents more of a financial model than a clinical model.

There are effective, ethical chiropractors. Make sure you see one if you choose this type of treatment. Your family doctor may know one near your home or office. Seek out that referral discussion or use someone who has helped a friend. Avoid the pre-paid programs and the like.

Massage

Massage therapy is more accepted in Europe than the US, and to my understanding, is far more in depth over the pond. This is another field with a wide variety of training backgrounds, skill sets, and cost structures. However, I do refer quite regularly to a small coterie of massage, cranio-sacral, and neuromuscular therapists in my community who I have come to know and trust.

One reason to get this treatment is relief of acute pain or injury. It can be hard to get that first PT appointment set up. Sometimes you can get massage therapy or body work arranged more quickly. Another factor is the hands-on healing element. Some of these practitioners have great manual skills to help your body release (fascia, muscles) and start healing. As with other treatments, if you are getting only temporary relief or the effects are diminishing, it may be time to reassess the appropriateness of the treatment or the practitioner for that problem.

Indigenous Medicine

Indigenous medicine is fascinating. In one culture, diagnosis is made by very careful tongue examination. In another, pulse diagnosis plays an important role. Studies and anecdotal reports have demonstrated that patients who are often immigrants from a particular society, may fail to benefit from Western medicine until they also incorporate a traditional healer's methods and approaches. Again, integrative care may provide the best of both.

Doctor's Note: *I'm open to complementary approaches that help my patients—acupuncture, chiropractic, massage—when used appropriately. But beware of expensive programs, unproven herbs, and treatments that go on indefinitely without results. Effective therapy should show benefits within a reasonable timeframe.*

CHAPTER 32
THE PREOPERATIVE EXAMINATION

If you ever need to have elective surgery, or even a medical procedure, you may be asked by your surgeon or proceduralist, to have a preoperative or medical clearance examination.

Purpose

The surgeon wants to make sure you are healthy before doing elective surgery. Elective is defined as non-emergency and can be important surgery like a gallbladder operation, or a hip replacement. While cosmetic or plastic surgery is almost always elective, it is a small percentage of the overall number of procedures for which an exam may be appropriate.

The anesthesiologist also wants to make sure you are healthy and understand any medical conditions you may have that could affect the choice of or use of anesthetic agents. The anesthesiologist's job is to keep you alive and healthy, out of pain, and often asleep/unconscious during the operation or procedure.

The Evaluation

You make an appointment with your Family Doctor and typically the surgeon also sends a note indicating the procedure and what testing he recommends to your PCP. When this doesn't arrive, an experienced physician should readily know what to do depending on your age and health status. Obviously your Family Doctor should know your health conditions better than anyone else. Also remember that you are having an elective procedure. If for some reason you get a fever or flu the day before you are scheduled to have surgery, let the surgeon know. Typically the procedure is rescheduled.

Back to your family doctor, who will take a brief history and find out any concerns you have about the procedure. I've had a few situations where a patient asked me, at the preoperative exam, whether they really needed the surgery and if they could seek a second opinion. Sometimes I've been able to clarify the necessity or alleviate their concerns.

Next I will check in on their health status of late, and update any medications they are taking, supplements, or medication allergies. I may emphasize stopping any aspirin a week before the procedure and avoiding many supplements, especially if they have a blood thinning property. Vitamin E, garlic, and fish oils may have this effect, usually benign or helpful, but not before surgery. Best to stop supplements a week before, but continue taking your prescription medication, usually until the morning of the surgery. Sometimes you'll be told to take morning meds with a sip of water, other times defer until after surgery.

Testing

After a fairly complete physical exam, blood tests should be drawn (or ordered). These typically include (see Laboratory chapter) a complete blood count, chemistry panel, sometimes a urine analysis and occasionally a blood clotting panel (PT/PTT tests cover this). Sometimes a surgeon will request other blood testing.

For patients above age 40 or 50 (depending on health status, hospital criteria, etc.) an electrocardiogram (EKG) may be performed by my assistant.

For patients with cardiopulmonary disease or above age 50 or 55, a chest x-ray is a reasonable part of this assessment. If someone has respiratory issues or asthma, pulmonary function testing may be done.

There are requests from the surgeon and there is the discretion on the part of the Family Doctor to do what is necessary to be able to say that the patient is ready for surgery.

Medical Clearance

If someone is high risk I'll probably have them see a cardiologist and/or other specialists prior to making a final determination. It's always better to have more information and more input when there are questions about this. Someone with a recent heart attack, for example, should generally not have elective surgery. Each health condition is individually evaluated before making a risk determination or "clearance" decision.

Doctor's Note: *Preoperative examinations are often necessary before you have surgery (and anesthesia). Your Family Doctor can typically do the exam and coordinate and review the laboratory and imaging that may also be needed. The testing is individualized based upon your age and health status.*

SECTION 7

Navigating Healthcare and Life Stages

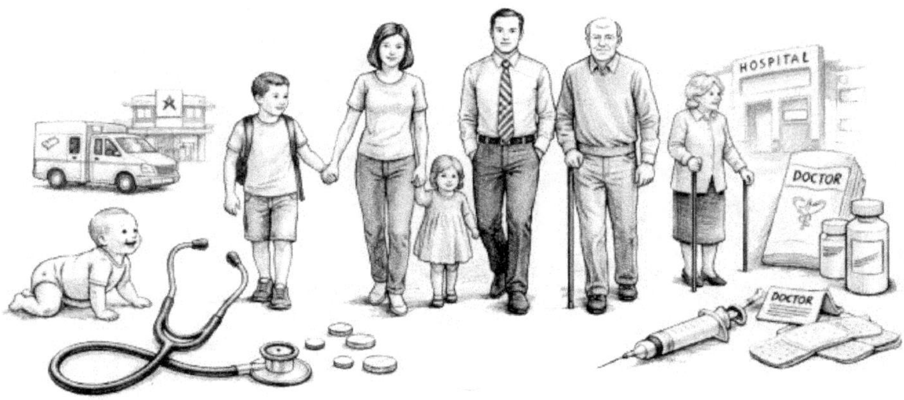

CHAPTER 33
NAVIGATING THE HEALTHCARE SYSTEM

Our healthcare system is complicated. PPO, HMO, preauthorization, online pharmacy, mail order pharmacy, delivery pharmacy, physical therapy at home, telehealth, urgent care, emergency room, primary care, specialty care, health insurance, Medicare. It goes on and on. I honestly believe that most physicians find the healthcare insurance system more complicated to learn than the vast amount we learn in medical school!

Over time, however, the physician (and his staff) does become an expert on the US healthcare system. I've even learned a lot about healthcare in Canada, Mexico, and parts of Europe. It is confusing. So helping my patients with the system and helping them to manage and reduce their costs is an important part of my job, as I see it. I note that many physicians are completely oblivious to patient costs and either ignore it completely or ask staff to deal with this area exclusively. As a family doctor, I've always been interested in helping my patients with the system and costs, and I'm a frugal person myself, so that helps.

Types of Health Insurance

Where to start? This chapter could be an entire book or online video course, by itself. Let's start with PPO, HMO, self-pay, Medicare, and Medicaid. PPO or preferred provider organizations are a mechanism for insurance companies to make available a network of physicians, in different specialties, to a patient/subscriber. Larger PPOs may have a broad network of doctors; smaller PPOs may have a more narrow network. This is something to think about when you're signing up for health insurance.

In addition, I try to give patients plenty of ways to see an in-network physician, where at all possible. The two main ways I do that are to provide a spreadsheet or part of a spreadsheet to my patients, via the secure portal, for any referrals. I send this by quickly typing and sending on the computer, while they are still in the office (or on the televideo). In addition, or where this list may not have the PPO doctors they need, I advise them to check their insurance plan directory, under a particular specialty, and choose a physician who is in-network. I instruct them to ask the office when they call, because any resource in my office or online may be out of date when it comes to physicians' participating status with any insurance company.

In-Network, Out-of-Network

Yes, it's complicated. I was an in-network physician for most of my career with most major PPO plans and Medicare. In the last few years I have moved away from that model and am out of network with most plans, in network with a few, and self-pay for most patients. Reimbursement is fee for service and is according to a pre-arranged or "negotiated" schedule, which differs from one PPO plan to another, and may vary from one physician or physician group to another. Regardless of what the physician's charges are, the patient is, at most, responsible for the approved rate. There may be a co-pay or deductible involved. A co-pay is paid at each visit, $20 to $50 usually; a deductible is from the beginning of the year until you pay off the $500 to $5000 deductible. In some cases, deductibles are waived for office visits or primary care visits.

Self-Pay

What is self-pay and how does it differ from a cash patient? The term "cash patient" has traditionally meant, in many medical offices, that you don't have health insurance or the doctor or patient is not in the same PPO or HMO network. It does NOT mean the patient is paying with twenty-dollar bills, although a minutely small number may do so. It just means that you are directly responsible to pay your bill, usually at the time of service, although some offices may bill you and ask you to pay within thirty days. Self-pay is very common among the psychotherapists I refer to. Self-pay is common among plastic surgeons for elective procedures. Self-pay is common among psychiatrists in my community.

So what are the major PPO plans? Anthem, also known as Blue Cross. Blue Shield, which in some states, is merged with Blue Cross as the "Blues". United Healthcare (UHC), Aetna, Cigna, Humana, PHCS are some others. Smaller plans are First Health and others.

HMO

What is an HMO? The term refers to Health Maintenance Organization. But the structure is the important distinction with the PPO model. In the HMO model, the primary care physician is often capitated. This means the doc is paid a monthly fee to be your doctor, whether you see him or not. There may be a co-pay, in addition, for an office visit. The doctor may be paid for some other services, but not usually. Obviously this produces a disincentive to actually see a patient in the office. More matters in HMO care tend to be handled via portal, email, telephone or office assistants. Usually a patient needs to see the primary care physician first, in an HMO plan, to get referrals to specialists and physical therapy and the like. While this can happen in PPO, it is usually not required. A person in a PPO can usually directly self-refer to a dermatologist for example. This might require a written authorization in HMO care. Specialists must be in the HMO network, as must imaging centers, and hospitals.

Another type of HMO is a closed panel model, the most well known of which is Kaiser Permanente, which started in California. In this environment, the physicians in the HMO are employees of the medical group, see patients in the HMO office building, and are paid a salary. They have less incentive, in theory, to do surgery or unnecessary procedures. They may even receive discipline about overuse of services. HMO plans tend to be good on preventive medicine and vaccinations and are not always as liberal with visits to physical therapy or psychotherapy, although this may vary. While you are in this model, you can see other physicians outside of the HMO but you are a self-pay in their office.

Medicare

Medicare is the national health system for those sixty-five and over. It also has a smaller number of participants who have been determined to be disabled, at a younger age, for at least a year, or permanently. Medicare covers 80% of the Medicare rate at the doctor's office or hospital. Many patients purchase a private plan (medigap policy) to cover the remaining 20% of the fee. Note that the rate is federally determined each year. Medicare has a small deductible at the beginning of the year which may be out of pocket and has some restrictions, such as twenty-four PT sessions a year, but is otherwise quite comprehensive.

There are also Medicare Advantage plans that may limit the doctors you can see, but offer more benefits at the same cost to you. For example, some offer a gym membership, eye glasses, or other benefits.

Medicaid

Medicaid is a nationally funded, state administered (in California, called Medi-Cal) system to provide care for poorer patients. This includes children, pregnant women, and those below a certain income level. Medicaid is often HMO or HMO-like and has a panel of physicians and other practitioners that you must see. Unfortunately, reimbursement is not great, and waiting times to see a specialist may therefore be longer. Medicaid has no deductible, and some patients find a good primary doctor in the system and stick with it as long as they are eligible. Clinics that do a lot of Medicaid care often have mid-level clinicians (nurse practitioners and physician assistants) provide a lot of the care to control costs.

Telehealth

Telehealth has been a boon. I recall when the pandemic emergency was called in 2020. The total shutdown I am referring to. I literally shifted, in one day, from seeing sixteen patients in the office to seeing sixteen patients the next day, via a telemedicine platform. It was a lifesaver for the patients and my practice. I learned the best ways to use the platform, and as we started seeing patients in the office again, my staff and I learned which patients needed an office visit and which might get perfectly adequate care online.

For example, someone who needed to be examined for a knee or sinus infection needed an office visit. Blood drawing, obviously in the office. If you had Covid, we might meet you in the parking lot for a swab, and then switch to telehealth from your car for the rest of your visit. When home Covid testing was available, we could do the whole visit from home. Mental health visits are quite appropriate for telehealth. The visit consists mostly of conversation. Refills of blood pressure medication could be done online, if the patient has an accurate cuff to give me a reading. If not, they needed to come in. An annual physical needed to be done in the office to examine the patient, draw blood, or do an EKG.

In-office visits remain the ideal, but telehealth can be useful for certain visits, as noted above, and save patients drive time, parking fees, etc.

Pharmacies

Prescribing medication to a pharmacy is really easy via my electronic health record. Just a few clicks. But getting the medication is not always that simple for my patient.

Sometimes the pharmacy is out of medication. This has been very common for certain medications since 2020, or even before. Attention deficit (ADHD) medications have, at times, been in limited supply. This necessitates sending a prescription later in the day or the next day, to another pharmacy, which is annoying, but necessary, duplicative work. Sometimes a "pre-authorization" is required. This means that the insurance company or pharmacy management component of the patient's healthcare insurance needs justification from the physician's office for the medication. For example, a testosterone level if you need to prescribe something to raise it. In a more extreme case, documentation of weight loss programs tried, for approval for a GLP-1 weight loss medication like Ozempic. This takes staff time, sometimes doctor time, and is not reimbursed. Sometimes my assistant can do this online, quickly; other times it takes phone calls and discussions with administrative people and is time consuming.

Pharmacies may also indicate that the patient can receive 90 days of a medication, whereas many prescriptions are only covered 30 days at a time. Ninety days makes a lot of sense for chronic medications, like blood pressure pills, that a patient is typically on for a long time. It makes no sense for a new medication where we don't know if it will be tolerated or effective. Sometimes we have to jump over this hurdle.

Hurdles and Hoops

Speaking of hurdles, it can be frustrating to feel like you are jumping over many hurdles and going through hoops to get your patient the care they need. The difficulty in getting this done eventually led me to completely stop seeing patients in the Workers' Compensation System. This system is notorious for denying care including medications and physical therapy. But on a daily basis, we deal with advanced imaging guidelines and associated hoops.

Let's say my patient comes in with a knee or shoulder injury. There are a few possibilities. The patient may really want an MRI (magnetic resonance imaging) scan to see what is structurally wrong (or not). I may desire the same MRI scan. If the injury is severe enough, for example, the knee is locked in a certain position or there is a massive swelling of the knee, it may be possible to get an MRI right away. However, usually, guidelines for imaging advise four weeks of MD-supervised conservative care which may include anti-inflammatory medications (NSAIDs) and physical therapy. So what do I advise? First of all, often it is quite reasonable and safe, sometimes effective, to do the medication and PT. But what if the patient insists or I have a higher level of concern? We can try getting authorization for the MRI, but this involves staff time, and often MD time for a "peer review". They can still deny the authorization.

A simpler solution, I have found, is to have a number of local MRI centers that offer a reasonable self-pay (or "cash") rate. MRI scans in my community can often be obtained for $300 to $350 for knee, shoulder, or back, without contrast being provided. For shoulders with injected contrast, maybe $500. Even the most expensive facilities often offer a self-pay rate below $600. Many patients, when informed of this, say, "I thought an MRI was $1000 or $2000." I respond that may have been the case years ago, but the self-pay rate now is often lower than the insurance rate.

How is this possible? When the patient uses insurance, it goes toward their deductible, which may be important in relation to the cost of other visits or surgery later in the year. If they pay out of pocket, they can use an FSA or HSA account if they have one (Flexible Spending Account, often provided by the employer or Health Savings Account, often self-financed as a tax deduction), which may allow them to use pre-tax earnings on healthcare. Again, my knowledge, and now your knowledge, can help navigate this complicated healthcare system and lower costs.

When it comes to authorizations, usually imaging centers will do that, for the patient's MRI or CT scan. For medications, our office can usually do the "prior authorization" and if approved, the medication is often covered, if needed, for a year.

Doctor's Note: *The healthcare system is confusing by design. Understanding PPOs, HMOs, deductibles, and workarounds can save you money and frustration. Don't hesitate to ask questions—navigating this maze is part of what your family doctor is here to help you with.*

CHAPTER 34

TECHNOLOGY AND HEALTH

A patient once came in and said, "Doc, I'm going to get this new device that measures all kinds of data, and I'm going to send you the data to review. I'm really excited by this!". My initial response, perhaps on a busy, busy day, was "Where will I get the time to review all this data, and who will pay me for the time to do so?"

I have become less cynical on this issue. First of all, I have found myself interested in wearable data. I wear an Apple Watch most days of the week and enjoy monitoring steps, heart rate during activity, and standing up time. I recently purchased an Ultrahuman ring and it is a great monitoring device (like the Oura ring) for sleep and other measurements. I purchased the Ultrahuman device through an online professional sales person, and he indicated that I could have a panel where I could see, with their consent, patient or family data.

This seemed to simplify the process of looking at data, and as the field grows and coalesces into a fewer number of companies, this may be more possible and more valuable. Detecting cardiac irregularities (like rhythm disturbances, atrial fibrillation, and the like), may be more convenient. I certainly find that home blood pressure data, which is currently only accurate on stand-alone arm-measuring devices, is helpful for managing patients who turn up with borderline data in the office.

Measure Blood Pressure at Home

I have advised people with borderline or elevated blood pressure, for years, to obtain a device for their personal use. These continue to improve and excellent brands include Omron, Hewlett Packard and Qardio. The capabilities of storing dozens of readings in the device's memory have been around for quite a while. In addition, newer devices upload data via Bluetooth to a phone and organize the data in tabular form which helps me when the patient returns to the office. Studies have shown a combination of office-measured data and home BP readings can help manage BP effectively.

Interestingly, some studies show that some patients read higher in the office, but some are actually higher at home. I try to get patients to bring their machine to an office visit so we can examine the accuracy of their sixty-dollar machine versus my one-thousand-dollar Welch Allyn device. Most are accurate, some are shockingly inaccurate and should be returned and a new one obtained.

It is still quite early in the wearable era, and I do not yet have experience reviewing patient data; I am still working on understanding my own sleep, stress, and recovery data on the Ultrahuman app! But I do anticipate these devices will have a myriad of benefits for patients and physicians. A key is good software—user friendly interfaces and design, and attention to making the data usable for the patient and the physician.

Collection vs. Insight

Some devices collect a lot of data. Is the information actionable? That is something we need to study and understand going forward. There may also be privacy concerns; read your agreements with these companies carefully. A lot more research needs to be done to determine how to help patient's health, with the data obtained by wearable devices.

Doctor's Note: *Wearable health tech can be valuable—but data alone isn't insight. Focus on devices that give you actionable information: blood pressure monitors, sleep trackers, heart rate monitors. Share meaningful patterns with your family doctor, not raw data dumps.*

CHAPTER 35

TRAVEL HEALTH

Patients of all ages, and stages in life, regularly have questions about travel medicine. There are now clinics that just specialize in this. Certainly for exotic locales, these clinics may be the only places to get unusual vaccinations. But for many travel locations, your family doctor is a great resource. Another amazing resource is the website www.cdc.gov/travel, which has general advice and country-specific advice. This is used by the public and healthcare professionals all the time.

Travel medicine depends almost entirely on where you are going. For example, North America (US, Canada)—sunscreen, mosquito repellent, tick advice, flu shot in the fall, Covid booster if you need one, stay hydrated on the plane; that's about all.

Mexico and Central and South America—some countries may have malaria and I check the CDC website for this. Malaria pills can be prescribed by your family doctor and making an accurate choice and advising how to take them is important. The CDC website helps. Dosing often involves starting before you arrive at the destination and may need to continue after you leave for maximum safety. Along with malaria medications, would be mosquito repellent and sometimes bed netting. Note that mosquitoes mostly avoid elevations above 6500 feet. Air conditioning may help as well.

Hepatitis A Shot(s)

Hepatitis A vaccination is recommended for many countries around the world. This is ideally a two-shot series and any travel vaccine should ideally be given at least two weeks before leaving. But sometimes you give it closer to departure, and there is some benefit of even one shot. The vaccine is good for at least five years. Hepatitis A is transmitted by contaminated water, ice cubes, glasses, poor hand-washing, etc.

Hepatitis B is transmitted by sexual contact, needles and the like, so typically not a risk for a couple traveling, but if you're single and may partake, make sure you are up to date.

Dengue fever is found in warmer countries and tropical areas. Mosquito repellent is key as there is currently no widely recommended vaccine. Treatment is supportive for this viral infection, also called "breakbone" fever. Flu-like symptoms, severe achy pains.

Western Europe, generally as safe as North America. Japan and Scandinavia, safer than the US! For some cities or regions, you may benefit from bottled water, as is advisable in Mexico and Central America, most of South America. For example, Venice, Italy, with a high water table, can have contamination. Drink bottled or boiled water. Some rural locations in Southern Europe, the same applies. Be cautious and stay healthy. GI illness is typically far from fatal, but very annoying and takes days to fully recover from, best to avoid where possible.

In some circumstances, we can prescribe medication to take at the first sign of symptoms or even prior to, when traveling to higher risk areas.

A polio booster is recommended for some countries. This is an injectable vaccine. The inactivated version is used.

A tetanus booster (Tdap) if it has been ten years, is always a good idea. Also covers pertussis (hence the P).

There is a typhoid vaccine (injectable or oral versions). Not incredibly effective, but again, applies to areas with questionable water, those that eat street food, etc.

As you can see, there is a lot of individualization for travel health. The basics apply to everyone: get up to date on your vaccinations, wear sunscreen and protective clothing, use mosquito and tick repellent. But a detailed review with your doctor can ensure you're prescribed medications for malaria prevention where appropriate, along with other region-specific recommendations. Plan in advance and budget for this consultation as part of preparing for big trips like an African safari or travel into rural Asia. Many countries have decent urgent care and emergency facilities, especially in big cities, and many doctors speak English adequately—some have even been trained in the US or UK. But prevention is always better than treatment abroad!

Travel Insurance

Obtaining travel insurance prior to a big or distant trip may be useful for some people. The benefits may be financial if you have to cancel a trip due to illness. But, depending on the plan you choose, the insurance company may also help coordinate your healthcare in other countries or even have the ability to medically evacuate you if you become seriously ill. Something to consider, especially for those who are older or who have chronic illness. Reminder: anyone can get appendicitis and there are countries where an operation would be quite safe and there are areas where this would not be the case.

> **Doctor's Note:** *Travel health is about preparation. Get your vaccines updated, know your destination's specific risks, and get prescriptions for preventive medications like malaria prophylaxis when needed. A 15-minute planning visit with your doctor can prevent weeks of misery on your trip. Consider travel insurance.*

CHAPTER 36

FAMILY PLANNING

I regularly get asked by male patients to check their sperm count. They may be concerned about fertility. This is an easy test to order, although the patient cannot just go to an ordinary lab. They need to go to a specialized lab that can examine sperm and create an accurate and usable report. Patients are advised by these centers to abstain for three days and either bring in a fresh specimen or produce one at the facility.

Do my male patients need to do this? I generally say no, unless they have not succeeded with a pregnancy after 6–12 months of trying. Usually over 35 years of age, six months merits an evaluation. Under 35, twelve months is typically reasonable. About 30% of infertility is caused by the man—low sperm count or poor quality of sperm. Women have a more complicated reproductive system and hence a higher percentage of infertility is caused by women's issues. I let a gynecologist address this, or a fertility specialist.

This also relates to another question I get from male patients. What do I need to do to increase the chance of a healthy baby? For a man, the biological process is simpler. Primordial sperm stem cells .... Ultimately sperm, ejaculation, fertilization. But, keeping your body as healthy as possible makes sense. Avoid substances for a few months like marijuana and non-prescribed drugs. Drink alcohol moderately, if at all. Eat well, and consider everything you put into your body as contributing, in a small way, to your sperm quality, quantity, and your ultimate success in fertilizing a healthy pregnancy.

The bottom line on family planning: it's more complicated for women than their male partners, so I advise women to see an OB-GYN for detailed pre-pregnancy recommendations. For my male patients, I recommend a common-sense approach—avoid substances like marijuana and non-prescribed drugs for a few months, drink alcohol moderately if at all, and remember that everything you put into your body contributes to sperm quality and quantity. When sperm testing is appropriate, I'll order a full analysis, but remember that these results aren't definitive. You can have a low sperm count and still achieve pregnancy, or have a great count and still face challenges—fertility depends on both partners. If you haven't conceived after 6–12 months of trying, that's when we start investigating further.

Vasectomy is probably the simplest permanent form of sterilization and my male patients often ask me about it after their second or third child, and sometimes with no children. I explain that the procedure must be considered permanent although a percentage can be reversed through complex microsurgery. The procedure itself is fairly simple, and in small communities, many family doctors have been trained in, and do this procedure. In major cities, a urologist is the doctor who typically does this procedure. It can be done under local or general anesthesia. The latter is my preference. I do emphasize that they will be asked challenging questions by the surgeon, in advance of the procedure. These questions relate to the possibility they would want to have additional children if they were to divorce, or if the tragedy of losing a child occurred. These difficult issues must be considered when contemplating permanent sterilization.

Often men get the procedure on a Friday, rest the weekend, and return to work Monday or Tuesday. Usually Tylenol or NSAIDs and an ice pack is all that is needed post-operatively, along with some rest. Wives are typically very indulgent of a husband who does this procedure (they won't need to take contraceptive pills any more) and watching TV on the couch is a great recovery activity for that weekend. Men can, of course, be apprehensive about this procedure. One uncommon option: friends scheduling this for the same day and getting a hotel room in which to order room service and relax, away from young children, for the weekend.

Doctor's Note: *Fertility concerns affect both partners. Simple testing can identify male factors, but give it time, 6–12 months of trying is normal. For complex issues, specialists in Reproductive Medicine offer the most advanced options.*

CHAPTER 37

Workplace Issues

There are a couple of major work-related issues that I've dealt with during my career as a family doctor. One is Workers' Compensation (Work Comp) injuries. These are injuries that occur to an employee at a company and are covered under a particular employer-carried health plan. This varies state by state, but is often a highly inconvenient type of care to obtain. Companies can insist that the patient see a particular doctor or clinic for care, although some will allow you to see your Family Doctor, especially if you have predesignated that doctor to provide care for Work Comp injuries. There may be many restrictions on getting imaging or even physical therapy through this type of insurance.

Injuries

Injuries may be physical injuries like lifting at work causing a back strain or shoulder injury. Injuries can also be psychological, like work stress emanating from a challenging supervisor. For physical injuries, physical therapy is often approved, medications, and some visits. The employer is allowed to see these records, and there may be pressure to return the injured employee to work quickly. Again, this may vary by state or region.

Stress and psychological issues are even more complicated, and documentation in all these matters is very important. In the last five to eight years, I have discontinued any involvement in Workers' Compensation, finding it to be a nuisance kind of medicine where there is a lot of paperwork and a lot of challenges in getting my patient the care they need, such as a longer course of physical therapy, imaging, or a specialist consultation. Many of these patients would get better care using their private health insurance, although there are sometimes laws that prevent this for work-related injuries.

Disability

The other issue that I continue to deal with related to work is a patient telling me they would like to "go on disability" at work. They need to stop working. They need a break. This often is related to stress at work or a clash with a supervisor or more rarely a co-worker. Most companies and states have provisions for disability. A physician typically is the one who must examine, diagnose, and document the reason for the disability and the duration.

I might give someone 2–4 weeks off work in these circumstances and reexamine them in the office. But before I do this, I have a frank discussion about disability and what the goals of the time off are. I have found, through experience, that time off work doesn't solve the underlying problem(s) at work. The patient/employee must decide if what is best for them is to change jobs or leave the company entirely. Sometimes the company may be flexible to keep an important worker; often the disability process alienates the company and the worker will eventually need to leave, anyway. Patients often benefit from counseling or therapy during the time off. Companies may have Employee Assistance Programs (EAPs) that provide four to six free sessions with a confidential therapist. Otherwise, patients can be referred to a private practice therapist, and I do so.

The key message about workplace health issues: whether you're dealing with a physical injury or psychological stress, proper documentation and honest communication with your doctor is essential. Workers' Compensation, while legally designed to protect you, often creates bureaucratic challenges that can delay care.

Disability leave can offer breathing room, but in my experience, time off alone rarely resolves the underlying workplace conflicts. During your time away, use therapy or counseling to gain clarity about whether to return to your job, request workplace modifications, or transition to a new position entirely. Your health—mental and physical—should never be sacrificed for any job.

Doctor's Note: *Workplace injuries—physical or psychological—deserve proper care, but Workers' Compensation can be frustrating. Disability leave can provide a needed break, but it rarely solves the underlying problem. Consider therapy and honest self-assessment about whether the job is right for you.*

CHAPTER 38

CAREGIVER SUPPORT

Sometimes my patients are in a situation where they have to provide care for a sick loved one. Someone with cancer or a spouse with progressive dementia. These are very challenging situations for the caregiver (and the person who receives the care).

Taking the perspective of the caregiver's doctor, I encourage them to get help, take breaks, take care of themselves as well as others, and utilize community and social services that may be available. Everyone gets the analogy from airplanes, "Put your oxygen mask on yourself before you put it on the child or elderly person next to you." Exercise and nutrition are important for the caregiver. Rest is crucial.

Respite care is a concept where the caregiver arranges for another family member, a paid individual, or a facility to take care of the loved one for a day, a week, or longer, to allow a break from caregiving. Some insurance plans provide support in this regard.

Finding the resources is something I try to help with. The patient must ultimately make the phone calls and commit to caring for themselves as well as their loved one. I try to advocate for my patient, listen to their issues, and be a problem solver and a support. It is certainly a challenging area of medicine.

Local and national resources include Alzheimer's Association, AARP, National Institute on Aging, Eldercare Locator and many more. American Cancer Society, Wellness Community, and other cancer focused organizations can be helpful, as well. There is the

United Way and many religious organizations (Catholic, Jewish, Christian) that are typically offering services to those of any or no faith.

Doctor's Note: *Caregivers often neglect their own health while caring for others. You can't pour from an empty cup. Accept help, take breaks, and remember that taking care of yourself isn't selfish—it's essential for sustaining your ability to care for your loved one.*

CHAPTER 39

END-OF-LIFE PLANNING

Ideally, this type of planning should occur way before a terminal illness and before one is elderly. If you are doing a will or trust with your attorney, that can be a time to put some words in writing about your wishes for a durable power of attorney for healthcare (e.g. a spouse or sister), living will, etc.

As a doctor, I should also be asking patients starting at age 60 or 65, if they have thought about end-of-life planning and the key documents mentioned above. But it's more than just documents. Expressing to their next of kin, their children, their loved ones, their wishes and desires about end-of-life care is extremely important. Talking about it with your family doctor is also important.

Sure, this is vitally important for a nursing home patient, or someone with cancer. But it is also important to understand your patient's preferences when it comes to artificial respiration, prolongation of life versus quality of life, etc. in other circumstances. Sometimes, catastrophic things occur suddenly. So take some time to think about this, discuss it with your closest family or friends and make decisions. Note that you can change your mind in the future. Your decisions and beliefs are not permanent, but they are important.

Doctor's Note: *End-of-life planning isn't morbid—it's a gift to your loved ones. Have the conversation early, write down your wishes, and update them as life changes. This removes the burden from your family during the most difficult times and ensures your values are honored.*

SECTION 8

Bibliography and Resources

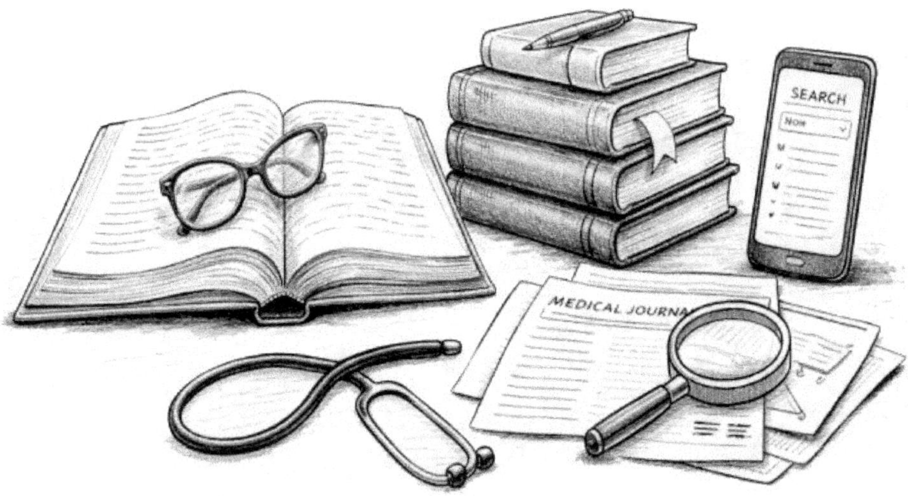

Selected Bibliography and Resources

BOOKS:

Schechter, David. Think Away Your Pain. MindBody Medicine Publications, 2014.

Sinclair, David A. Lifespan: Why We Age—and Why We Don't Have To. Atria Books, 2019.

Attia, Peter. Outlive: The Science and Art of Longevity. Harmony, 2023.

Walker, Matthew. Why We Sleep. Scribner, 2017.

MEDICAL REFERENCES:

Cancer Screening:

- Klein EA, et al. Clinical validation of Galleri multi-cancer detection test. *Annals of Oncology*. 2021.
- National Cancer Institute. www.cancer.gov

Cardiovascular Health:

- American Heart Association/American College of Cardiology Cholesterol Guidelines. *Circulation*. 2019.
- Lincoff AM, et al. SELECT Trial: Semaglutide and cardiovascular outcomes. *New England Journal of Medicine*. 2023.
- Cholesterol Lowering goals: Grundy SM, Stone NJ, Bailey AL, et al. 2018 AHA/ACC/AACVPR/AAPA/ABC/ACPM/ADA/AGS/APhA/ASPC/NLA/PCNA Guideline

on the Management of Blood Cholesterol. *Circulation.* 2019;139(25):e1082-e1143.

Weight Management:

- Lincoff AM, et al. Semaglutide and Cardiovascular Outcomes in Obesity. *NEJM.* 2023.

Supplements:

- Age-Related Eye Disease Study 2 (AREDS2). *JAMA.* 2013.
- National Eye Institute: www.nei.nih.gov/areds2

Mental Health:

- Kroenke K, Spitzer RL, Williams JB. The PHQ-9 depression screener. *Journal of General Internal Medicine.* 2001.
- PHQ-9 questionnaire: www.phqscreeners.com
- Kessler RC, et al. Adult ADHD Self-Report Scale. *Psychological Medicine.* 2005.
- ASRS screener: www.hcp.med.harvard.edu/ncs/asrs.php

Chronic Pain:

- Apkarian AV, et al. Chronic pain and brain structure changes. *Journal of Neuroscience.* 2004.
- Schechter D. *Think Away Your Pain.* MindBody Medicine Publications, 2014.

PATIENT RESOURCES:

- American Academy of Family Physicians: www.aafp.org
- Centers for Disease Control and Prevention: www.cdc.gov
- National Institutes of Health: www.nih.gov
- Chronic Pain: www.neuroplastic.org
- Chronic Pain: www.mindbodymedicine.com
- Travel Medicine: www.cdc.gov/travel

TOPIC FINDER

Note to Readers:
This Topic Finder is organized alphabetically by subject.

Numbers refer to **chapters**, not page numbers. Some topics are discussed in more than one chapter.

A
Abdominal pain—17
ABCDE rule for skin lesions—22
Acid reflux—17, 29, 30
Acupuncture—31
ADD / ADHD—30
Adderall—30
Advanced directives—39
Advil—16, 29
Aging—9, 10, 11, 12, 27, 28, 39
Albuterol—26, 30
Alcohol use—1, 2, 3, 4, 7, 17, 23, 29, 35
Allergies—1, 18, 29, 30
Alternative medicine—31
Alzheimer's disease—8, 9, 34
Amitriptyline—10, 30
Amlodipine—30
Amoxicillin—18, 19, 20, 30
Ankle injuries—5, 16
Antibiotics—18, 19, 20, 29, 30
Antidepressants—23, 30
Anti-aging—9
Anxiety—2, 14, 15, 23, 30
Aspirin—7, 29, 30, 32
Asthma—26, 30, 32, 35
Atherosclerosis—7
Atorvastatin—7, 30
AUTO-PAP—10

B
B12 supplementation—12, 30
Back pain—13, 16, 29, 30, 31, 37
Behavioral health—13, 14, 23
Bell curve and lab results—3
Benzodiazepines—10, 30
Bilirubin—3
Biopsychosocial model—1, 13, 14, 23

Bladder infection—19
Blood pressure—2, 3, 7, 24, 30, 34
Blood sugar—3, 11, 24, 30
Blood tests—3, 6, 7, 8, 11, 12, 24, 25, 28, 32
Blue Zones—9
BMI—2, 11, 24
Bone density—6, 27
Bone health—12, 27, 28
BRCA genes—8
Breast cancer screening—6
Bronchitis—18, 26, 29
Bupropion—23, 30

C
Calcium score—7
Calcium supplements—12, 27, 29
Cancer screening—6, 8, 22
Carbohydrates—4, 11, 24
Cardiac CT angiogram—7
Cardiac prevention—7
Cardiovascular disease—2, 3, 4, 5, 7, 11, 24, 30
Caregiver support—38
Chlamydia—20
Cholesterol—3, 4, 7, 24, 30
Chronic cough—18, 26
Chronic pain—13, 14, 16, 23, 29, 30, 31
Colds—18, 29
Colon cancer screening—6
Colonoscopy—1, 6
Common prescription medications—30
Complete blood count / CBC—3, 32
COPD—26, 30, 32
Coronary artery disease—7
COVID-19—18
CPAP—10
Creatinine—3, 32
CT angiogram—7
CT scan—2, 7, 13, 16, 33

D
Depression—14, 23, 30, 37
Diabetes—3, 11, 24, 30
Diet—2, 4, 7, 11, 17, 24
Digestive health—17
Disability leave—37
Diverticulitis—17
Doctor-patient relationship—Introduction, 1, 2, 33
Doctor's Notes—Introduction
Doctor's visit preparation—1
Drug interactions—12, 29, 30, 32
Durable power of attorney—39

E
Ear, nose, and throat symptoms—2, 18, 29
Eczema—22, 29
EHR / electronic health record—1, 2, 33, 34
EKG / ECG—7, 32

Emergency room—1, 33
End-of-life planning—39
Erectile dysfunction—21, 28, 30
Escitalopram—23, 30
Exercise—1, 2, 5, 7, 9, 10, 11, 13, 16, 23, 24, 27, 38
Exercise injury—5, 16, 37
Eye examination—2

F

Family history—1, 3, 6, 7, 8, 24, 25
Family planning—36
Fasting—3, 4
Fatigue—10, 14, 23, 24, 25, 28, 30
Fertility—28, 36
Fever—18, 19, 26, 35
Fiber—4, 17
Fish oil—12, 29, 32
Flu—18, 29, 35
Flu vaccine—6, 18, 35
Food choices—4, 11, 17, 24
Food poisoning—17
Forms for doctor visits—1
Frozen shoulder—16
Full-body MRI—6, 14
Furosemide—30

G

Gabapentin—10, 13, 30
Galleri / MCED testing—6, 14
Genetic testing—8
GERD—17, 29, 30
Gilbert's syndrome—3
GLP-1 medications—2, 11, 24, 30
Glucose—3, 24
Gonorrhea—20
Gout—3, 16, 30
Grief—23, 38, 39

H

HbA1c—3, 24
Headaches—15
Health insurance—33, 35
Healthcare navigation—33
Healthcare technology—34
Heart attack prevention—7
Heart disease—3, 6, 7, 24, 30, 32
Heart rate—2, 7, 25, 30, 34
Heart scan—7
Hemoglobin—3
Hemoglobin A1c—3, 24
Hepatitis A—35
Hepatitis B—20, 35
Hepatitis C—20
Herpes—20
High blood pressure—2, 7, 24, 30, 34
Hip pain—16
HMO—33
Home blood pressure monitor—2, 34
Hormone therapy—28
Hormones—3, 21, 25, 28, 30
Hospice—39

Hyaluronic acid injections—16
Hypertension—2, 7, 24, 30, 34

I

Imaging—2, 6, 7, 13, 14, 16, 33
Immunizations—6, 18, 35
In-network care—33
Incidental findings—6, 7, 14
Injury avoidance—5
Insurance—33, 35
Intermittent fasting—4
Irritable bowel syndrome / IBS—17

J

Jet lag—10, 35
Joint injections—16
Joint pain—16, 29, 30
Joint replacement—16, 32

K

Kidney function—3, 19, 24, 30, 32
Kidney tests—3
Knee pain—16
Knee replacement—16, 32

L

Laboratory testing—3, 6, 7, 8, 11, 12, 24, 25, 28, 32
LDL cholesterol—3, 4, 7, 30
Levothyroxine—25, 30
Lifestyle—1, 2, 4, 5, 7, 9, 10, 11, 23, 24, 38
Lipid panel—3, 7
Lisinopril—30
Living will—39
Losartan—30
Low back pain—13, 16, 37
Lung disease—18, 26, 32

M

Malaria prevention—35
Mammography—6
MCED / multi-cancer early detection testing—6, 14
Medical clearance—32
Medical records—1, 33, 34
Medicare—33
Medication list—1, 29, 30, 32
Medication safety—29, 30, 32
Medications—1, 10, 12, 18, 19, 20, 21, 23, 24, 25, 26, 28, 29, 30, 31, 32
Mediterranean diet—4, 7, 11, 24
Melanoma—22
Melatonin—10, 29, 30
Menopause—28
Mental health—13, 14, 23, 37, 38
Metformin—24, 30
Metoprolol—30
Migraine—15, 30
Mind-body medicine—13, 14, 23, 31
Moles—22
MRI—2, 6, 13, 14, 16, 33

Muscle strengthening—1, 5, 9, 11, 27

N
Nasal congestion—18, 29
Nasal irrigation—18, 29
Neck pain—13, 16
Neuroplastic pain—13, 14, 23, 31
NSAIDs—16, 29, 30, 32
Nutrition—1, 4, 7, 11, 12, 17, 24, 38

O
Office visit—1, 2, 3
Omeprazole—17, 29, 30
Ophthalmoscope—2
Osteoarthritis—16, 27
Osteopenia—27
Osteoporosis—27, 28
Out-of-network care—33
Over-the-counter medications—29
Ozempic—11, 24, 30

P
Pain—13, 14, 16, 29, 30, 31
Pain management—13, 16, 29, 30, 31
Pantoprazole—17, 30
Patient history—1
Patient portal—33, 34
Patient preparation—1
Physical activity—1, 2, 5, 7, 9, 10, 11, 24, 27, 38
Physical examination—2, 32
Physical therapy—5, 13, 16, 31, 37
Pneumonia—18, 26
PPO—33
Prediabetes—3, 11, 24, 30
Prenuvo—6, 14
Preoperative examination—32
Prescription medications—30
Preventive care—2, 6, 7, 8
Primary care—Introduction, 1, 2, 6, 33
Probiotics—17
Prostate cancer screening—2, 3, 6
PRP / platelet-rich plasma—16
PSA test—2, 3, 6
Psychological stress—13, 14, 23, 37
Pulmonary function testing—26, 32

Q
Questions for your doctor—Introduction, 1, 2, 3, 6, 33
Quitting smoking—1, 7, 18, 26

R
Referrals—1, 2, 16, 22, 33
Reflux—17, 29, 30
Resistance training—1, 5, 9, 11, 27

Respiratory infection—18, 26
Respite care—38
RICE method—5, 16
Rosuvastatin—7, 30
Rotator cuff—16
RSV vaccine—6, 18, 35

S
Screening tests—6, 7, 8, 22, 27
Sciatica—13, 16
Self-pay medical care—33
Semaglutide—11, 24, 30
Sertraline—23, 30
Sexually transmitted infections—20
Shoulder pain—16
Sinus infection—18, 29, 30
Skin cancer—2, 22
Skin growths—22
Sleep—10, 11, 23, 30
Sleep apnea—10
Smoking—1, 7, 18, 26
Social history—1
Sperm count—36
SSRIs—23, 30
Statins—7, 30
Stem cell injections—16, 31
Stress—13, 14, 15, 23, 37, 38
Supplements—3, 9, 12, 29, 30, 31, 32
Surgery clearance—32
Syphilis—20

T
Telehealth—33, 34
Testosterone—3, 21, 28, 30
Thyroid disease—3, 25, 28, 30
Tirzepatide—11, 24, 30
Travel health—35
Travel insurance—35
Trazodone—10, 30
Triglycerides—3, 7, 24
Tylenol / acetaminophen—16, 29
Typhoid vaccine—35

U
Ultrasound—3, 16
Urgent care—18, 19, 33
Urinalysis—3, 19, 32
Urinary tract infection—19
Uric acid—3, 16
USPSTF—6

V
Vaccines—6, 18, 35
Vasectomy—36
Viagra—21, 30
Vital signs—2
Vitamin B12—12
Vitamin D—12, 27, 30
Vitamins—12, 29, 30

W
Waist circumference—2, 11, 24
Wearable technology—34

Weight management—2, 4, 11, 24, 30
Wegovy—11, 24, 30
Wellness—4, 5, 9, 10, 11, 12
White coat hypertension—2
Workplace issues—37
Workers' Compensation—37
Wrist pain—16

X

X-rays—2, 13, 16, 32, 33

Y

Yoga—5, 10, 13, 31

Z

Z-drugs—10
Zepbound—11, 24, 30
Zolpidem / Ambien—10

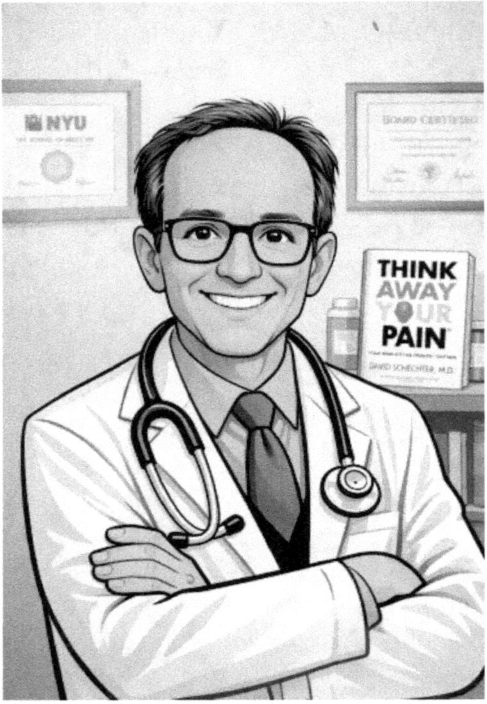

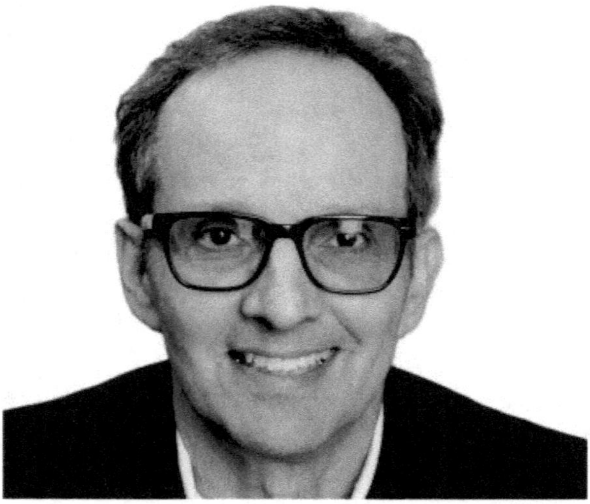

David Schechter, M.D.

www.ingramcontent.com/pod-product-compliance
Lightning Source LLC
LaVergne TN
LVHW022214200926
848481LV00006B/1967